TATTOOS OF I...

MAGIC, DEVOTION, & PROTECTION

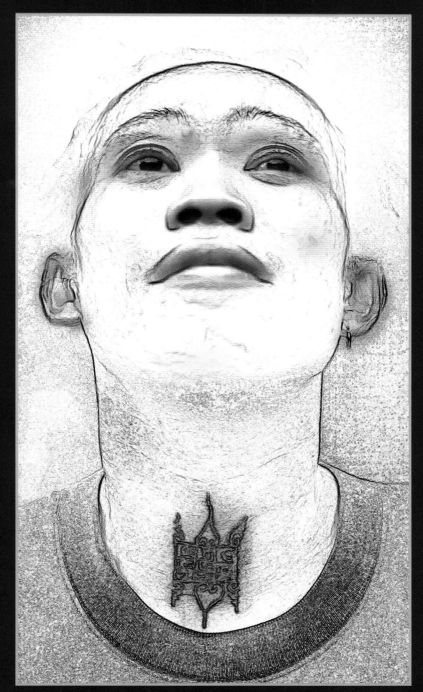

THAILAND, CAMBODIA, & LAOS

MICHAEL MCCABE

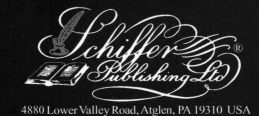

Schiffer Publishing Ltd

4880 Lower Valley Road, Atglen, PA 19310 USA

DEDICATION

For R.O. Tyler who introduced me
to the magic of tattooing.

Cover and book design by: Bruce Waters
Type set in Abaddon heading font/text font Korinna BT

ISBN: 0-7643-1679-6
Printed in China

Published by **Schiffer Publishing Ltd.**
4880 Lower Valley Road
Atglen, PA 19310
Phone: (610) 593-1777; Fax: (610) 593-2002
E-mail: Schifferbk@aol.com
Please visit our web site catalog at **www.schifferbooks.com**
We are always looking for people to write books on new and related subjects. If you have an idea for a book please contact us at the above address.

This book may be purchased from the publisher.
Include $3.95 for shipping.
Please try your bookstore first.
You may write for a free catalog.

In Europe, Schiffer books are distributed by
Bushwood Books
6 Marksbury Ave.
Kew Gardens
Surrey TW9 4JF England
Phone: 44 (0) 20 8392-8585; Fax: 44 (0) 20 8392-9876
E-mail: Bushwd@aol.com
Free postage in the U.K., Europe; air mail at cost.

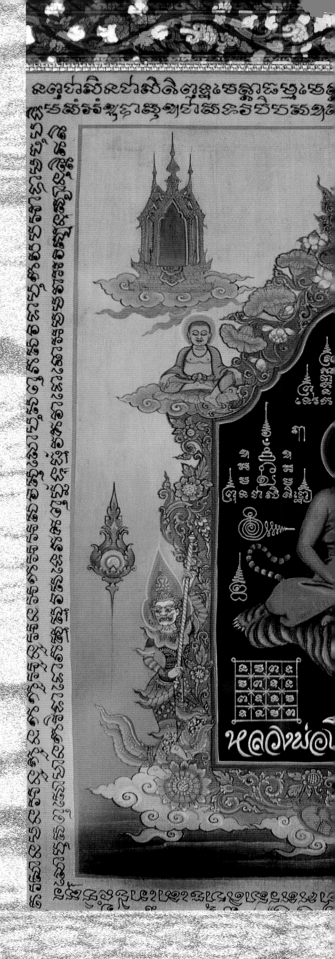

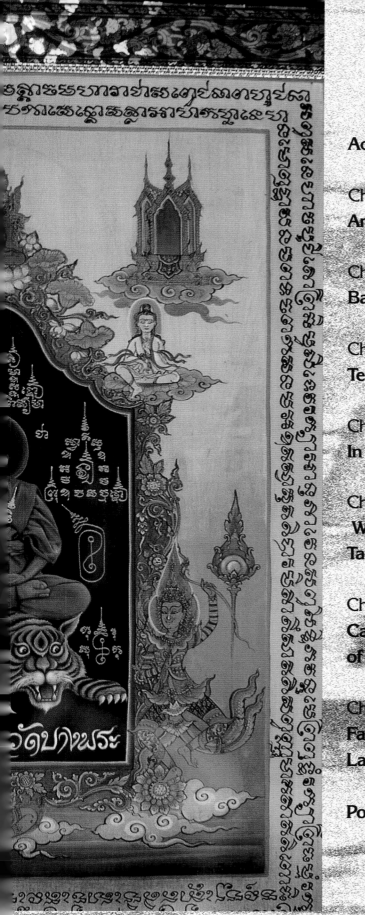

CONTENTS

Acknowledgments

Many people helped me to realize this project. It represents a departure from my work to date and the research took place in a challenging part of the world. First, I would like to thank Barbara Lee for her support throughout the process of creating this book. I would also like to thank Richard Guitard of Bangkok for his generosity and James Pate of Bangkok for his knowledge and insight.

In Bangkok, Thailand tattooers Jimmy and Joy Wong were very generous with their time and knowledge. Kevin and Keith Conley were also very helpful. Sukhumvit Road tattooer Amporn Klahan (Ouy) and her friends Rangsan Sinprasert (Pae) and Supannee Starojitski (Lee) helped a great deal. The folks at Larry's Dive on Soi 22, particularly Nok, were good friends, kept me well fed and took good care of me while I was in town.

In Chiang Mai, Thailand I would like to thank my Tuk-Tuk man Sammy who drove me a long way into the hills to meet his family and visit a remote tattoo temple. His generosity is greatly appreciated. I would also like to thank the members of the Chiang Mai Jungle Club for taking me along, deep into the jungle.

In Phnom Penh, Cambodia, I would like to thank Craig and Vibeke of Vibes Tattoo and Anna of *The Cambodian Daily* for their help introducing me to the tattoo magician, Kong Sengheurn. My motorbike taxi driver Chan was very loyal and I thank him for his mysterious late night tours of darkened Phnom Penh. In Siem Reap, Cambodia, I would like to thank my driver Ouy and the young kids at Angkor Wat who tiptoed me safely through a minefield into the jungle to the remote tattoo temple Bria Branom. I also would like to thank monk Mut.

In Laos, the Tuk-Tuk men of Vientiane were very generous, bringing me to their favorite restaurant hangout where I was well fed with home cooked, smoking-hot curries. After an exhausting 17-hour trek into the mountains, I am in debt to an anonymous young woman and her son who went out of their way very late one night in Luang Prabang, Laos, to make sure I had a safe place to stay. Thank you. I also wish to thank Seangphone, who took me to several temples in Luang Prabang where he had studied Buddhism as a boy. He introduced me to several senior monks and translated their insights about magical tattooing and Buddhism. Without his introduction and guidance, I would have been closed out of the opportunity to truly experience the roots of Lao tattoo.

Thanks to Wes Wood, Matty Jankowski, and the staff at Sacred Tattoo (NYC) for giving me an extended leave of absence to do this research. Also thanks to Kevin Craig for his help with information about the Hindu pantheon.

My appreciation to Jay Freedman and Beryl and Phil Gates for their interest and support of my work over the years.

Thank you to Alison Reilly for her expertise capturing still images from video shot in Bangkok.

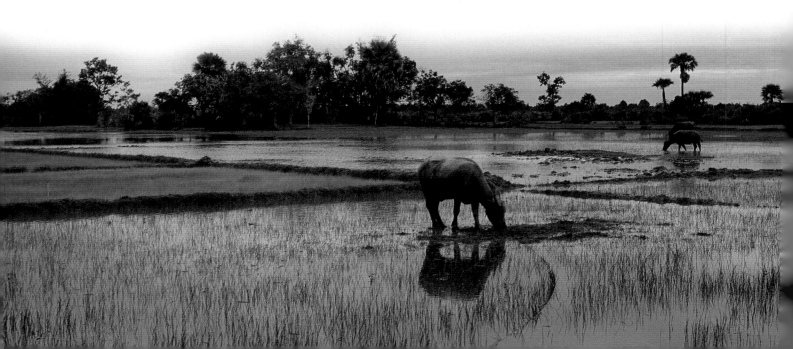

Chapter One

An Introduction

The #38 bus that crawls up the Bangkok street called Sukhumvit weaves through a sea of unforgiving, unflinching traffic. At the helm, the middle-aged driver with the patience of a saint keeps his left hand on the gearshift, poised for the unlikely possibility that he will have the opportunity to shift into second gear. It's as if his vessel were trapped in a school of fish; there's no place to go.

A thin, young woman with short hair makes her way along the wood plank floor of the bus. She is wearing a baggy, dark blue municipal uniform of cotton pants and a loose fitting button down shirt. The transit system logo patch on her pocket bobs along as she shuffles. She looks bored, and finally sits in an empty seat adjusting her protective white cotton facemask. It is oppressively hot in the bus, the windows are open and the gray, smoggy air is pushed by oscillating ceiling fans that twist around in a futile dance, their cooling task completely hopeless.

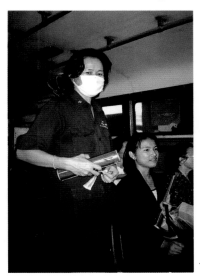

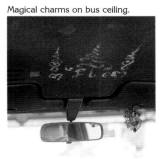

Magical charms on bus ceiling.

Ticket woman on Bangkok bus.

At the front of the bus, over the driver's head, there are a few magical charms crudely painted on the sheet metal ceiling. They have curlicue chedi or stupa-like shapes resting on a bed of sacred writing and are meant to protect the bus, the driver, the passengers, and the ticket taker who has risen to take fares from passengers who have just jumped on board — literally. The belief in protective, sacred charms and amulets runs deep in this part of the world. Across from the ticket woman, a man in his early forties is managing a catnap somehow. As his head bobs backwards to the rhythm of the bus's creep, tiny tattoo stupa symbols similar to the ones on the bus ceiling are revealed on his throat. They start just under his chin and run delicately down to his Adam's apple. There is ancient Khmer script framing the whole composition. Like the charms on the bus ceiling, these tattoo marks are meant to protect the man who wears them.

To an outsider, especially an occidental; the world that people in Indochina inhabit is neither sublime nor complex — it simply doesn't exist. Reality in this part of the world is pregnant with a maze of interacting belief systems including Buddhism, Hinduism, Animism, and ancestor worship that is very old, stretching back to ancient Khmer Kingdom times. It is difficult to summarize, but the variables of both waking and subconscious reality of many people living here, particularly traditionally based people, would be completely terrorizing for the western outsider. Reality in this part of the world is denser and full of options. Navigating through this type of nuanced world is risky and uncertain.

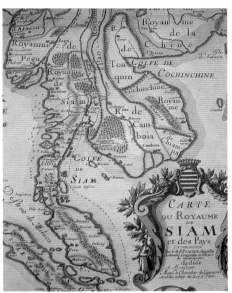

French colonial map of Indochina.

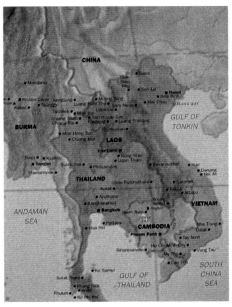

Map of Indochina.

Imagine approaching a traffic light at an intersection and finding it a hundred feet tall with not three lights but hundreds of them shining all different colors. Now image that you could control these lights to respond to a wish or command and the result could depend on the day of the week, the hour of the day, the month, the year; how you behaved yesterday, last week, last lifetime. Imagine that living in this type of complex reality was status quo and normal. This simple metaphor begins to crudely describe the arrangement of life for many in Indochina where most people worship dozens of deities, sacred objects, guardian spirits, and the spirits of former living heroes and heroines. The charms found on bus ceilings, storefronts, pieces of fabric and tattoos are diagrams that illustrate the possibility of controlling the uncertainty of life in some way.

Noom is thirty-seven years old and has tattooed since 1995. He works in the non-touristy Prakhanong section of Bangkok. He finds himself tattooing an assortment of contemporary images heavily inspired by Western pop culture, but he respects the traditional images and motivations of Thai and Khmer magical tattooing. Like many of his contemporaries, Noom has several magical tattoos located around his body. "Many people, young and old, in my neighborhood live in two worlds: the Old World of magic and superstition and a modern world influenced by the west," he explains.

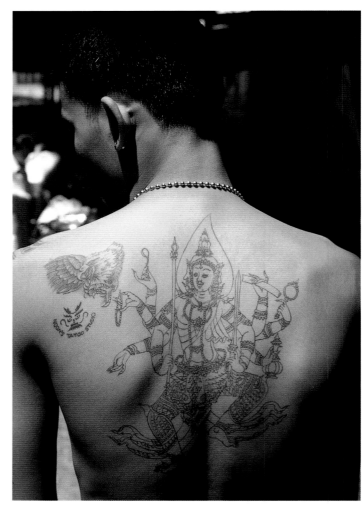

Magical tattoo on Noom's customer.

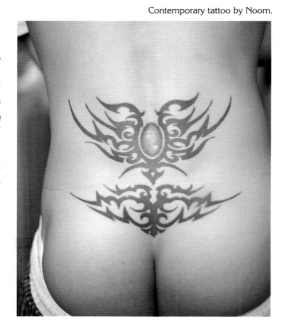

Contemporary tattoo by Noom.

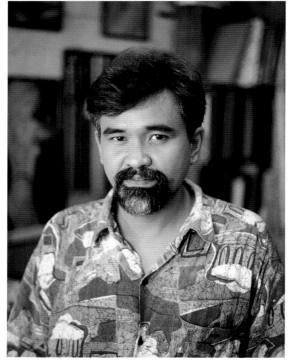

Bangkok tattooer, Noom.

"Many people, young and old, in my neighborhood live in two worlds: the Old World of magic and superstition and a modern world influenced by the west."

6

"A lot of people still believe in the old Khmer cults of ancestor worship. There are *Genji*, which are powerful spirits of nature, and there are *Neak-Ta* that are the ancestral spirits of the neighborhood or village. People associate them with things like the hills, the trees and rocks. These spirits are very powerful and they protect things.

Tattoos by Noon.

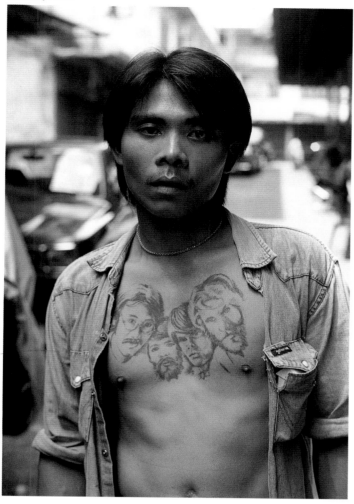

Magical tiger tattoo by Noom.

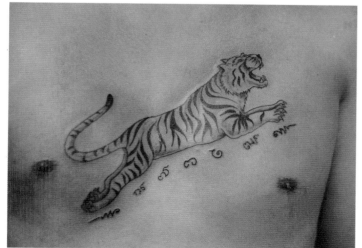

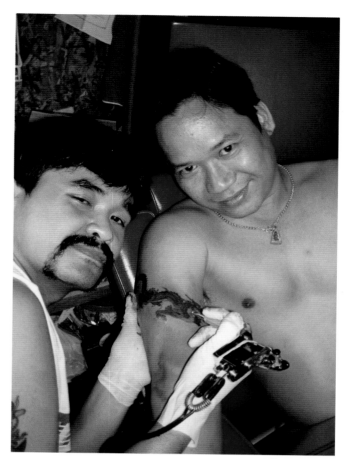

Noom tattooing.

"People in my part of the world are still very superstitious. They beg favors from spirits and Gods and if their wishes are granted they pay respect and make payments of some kind to the spirits. For example, there are small house lizards called *Jing-Joks* that people think bring good luck to the household. At night, the lizards make this 'Tch, tch' call and people think it is a warning of some kind. If you hear it when you leave the house, don't leave! If you hear the call before you do anything, don't do it! If the call comes from behind you it means you will have trouble from somebody who is jealous of you. If it comes from your left it means your efforts over the next few days will be successful. If it comes from your right you will experience some form of suffering.

Noom's customers.

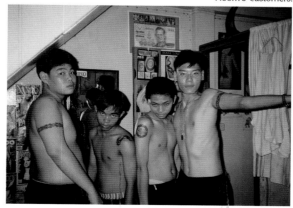

7

"I have friends who get their hair cut only on certain days. They think if you get your hair cut on a Sunday, it will bring you a long life. If you get it cut on a Monday it will bring you health and happiness. On a Tuesday it will bring you power. They never get their hair cut on Wednesday, it will bring you disaster! A lot of barbershops are closed on Wednesday. If you get it cut on Thursday, the Thevada or guardians will protect you."

Noom continues to explain some of the significance of Thai and Khmer tattooing.

"In the city, some families will not encourage putting spells on people. People in the country still believe in the old style tattooing that makes people look strong. *Sak* is the term used in this part of the world for a tattoo. *Poi-Sak* means on the body. A teacher or monk who tattoos is called an *Arjan-Sak*. Sometimes young people who get tattooed at a temple can identify others who have been tattooed there too. They can pick out the work of a particular monk and they identify with people who have had work done by the same Arjan. If they get into a fight but see the work of the same Arjan on a person, they will stop fighting them because they are in the same group. Each tattoo master has his own signature or mark called the *Yan Khu*. It is usually the first tattoo that is given to a new student on the neck, forearm or back of the hand. Those with the same mark avoid conflicts with each other and share in a kind of camaraderie.

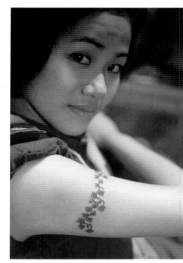

Noom's customer.

"Different Arjans specialize in their own skills and reputations. Some specialize in tattooing the tongue of women for good talking in business although the tattooing of women is rare. The specialized marks are called *Salika* and are named after a Mynah bird known for its alluring song. Men may tattoo the head to prevent accidents. A monk or a Wat (temple) may have a reputation for tattooing a tiger on the chest or an image of the monkey king Hanuman on the arm. He is the first body guard of Lord Rama and people like him because of his sincerity to protect his boss Lord Rama. The Khmer lion is tattooed as a symbol of strength. In the old days men were tattooed for protection when they went to war. Designs were put on clothing to be worn into battle for those who didn't want to get tattooed."

At the front of Noom's shop there is a framed mystical diagram hanging on the wall. The worn piece of paper has a central image of a sitting Buddhist monk surrounded by a geometric design that is made up of small quarter inch squares looking something like a newspaper crossword puzzle. Each square has a Khmer letter neatly penned in it and when all the letters are combined they represent a magical spell meant to produce good business. Geometric designs like this are part of tradition in Indochina that dates back beyond the time of Marco Polo.

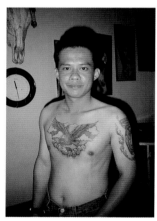

Noom's customers.

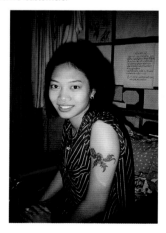

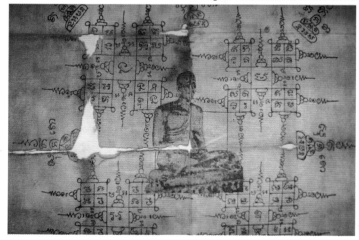

Magical charm in Noom's tattoo studio.

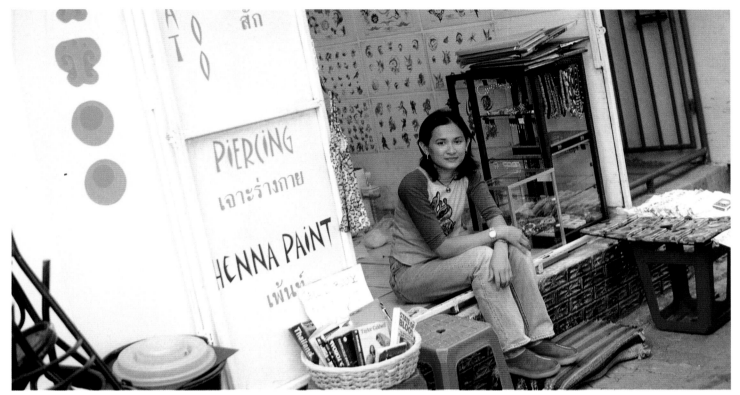

Ouy at her Sukhumvit tattoo booth.

A young woman whose nickname is Ouy tattoos on the notorious street called Sukhumvit in Bangkok. Her spotless, sidewalk level booth is open to the hectic street. Huge, belching busses, tuk-tuk taxis, and thousands of cars fly past a few feet from her small work area. Curious pedestrians stride past sneaking peaks at the modern tattoo flash she hangs neatly on her clean, white walls.

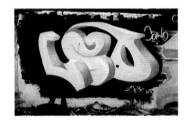 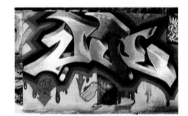

Graffiti near Ouy's tattoo booth.

Ouy

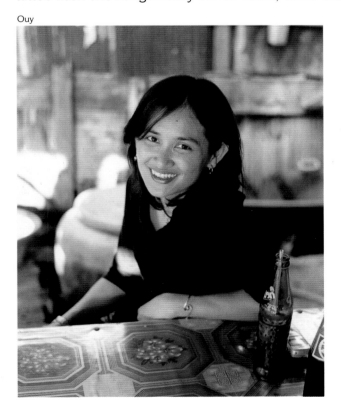

"When I tattoo modern style designs, I can pursue my interests in art. I can experiment with color, the design qualities. I can make things interesting for myself."

This is an adventurous move for a 29-year-old woman. Her section of Bangkok is infamous to say the least. The completely over-the-top streets called Soi Cowboy and Soi Nana, where half naked girls dance in seedy bars to the frantic Western beat, are a few feet away. Nightly she does battle with drunken foreigners, pickpockets, drug addicts, and streetwalkers. A lot for a pretty woman to deal with while she's trying to make a living.

She started to tattoo two years ago and has maintained her shop for just over a year. As a young woman in college she studied to become a secretary but quickly became disillusioned with that path. Her exhusband was an accomplished Bangkok tattooer and after they broke up, she decided to pursue the art to support herself and her young daughter.

9

In terms of the artwork, she likes modern tattoo designs more than the superstitious tattoo designs that are traditional to Thailand. "When I tattoo modern style designs," she comments. "I can pursue my interests in art. I can experiment with color, the design qualities. I can make things interesting for myself."

To be a tattoo businesswoman in Bangkok is challenging. There are no tattoo teachers so she had to learn it all on her own. She knows that her tattoo customers are looking for a tattooer who is very professional, knows the trade, and knows the ropes. She likes what she is doing but feels that this is the first step for her. She wants to improve her skill and ability as a tattoo artist, but realizes it will take time.

Tattooers in urban areas like Bangkok get an assortment of customers with sophisticated tastes that have been influenced by the global enthusiasm about tattooing. Tattoo magazines are everywhere, influencing what people want for tattoos. Ouy explains, "A lot of tourists come by my shop on their way to Soi Cowboy. They look at the pictures on my wall and choose one. They are the same pictures they could get at home, but they want a tattoo from Bangkok. They are happy to see me working in my booth. They like that I keep things very clean."

Like Noom, Ouy straddles the two tattoo worlds that coexist today in Indochina and respects them both. Her friend Pae (pronounced Pay) is approximately her age but does not necessarily embrace the new tattoo styles influenced by the West. His back and arms are heavily tattooed with exact, parallel rows of magical Khmer script that look like they have been applied with the exactness of a typewriter. He also has a few Hindu deities that are popular, traditional tattoo images. Pae has the image of an Indian hermit or *Ruesi* tattooed on him. These hermits appeared early in Indian mythology as intermediaries between humans and gods and they are worshiped by Arjan and devoted tattoo patrons. There are as many as 108 hermits but only a handful are identified by name as guardians of tattooing. Ruesi Narot is the incarnation of the Hindu god Vishnu and is honored by tattooers throughout Indochina.

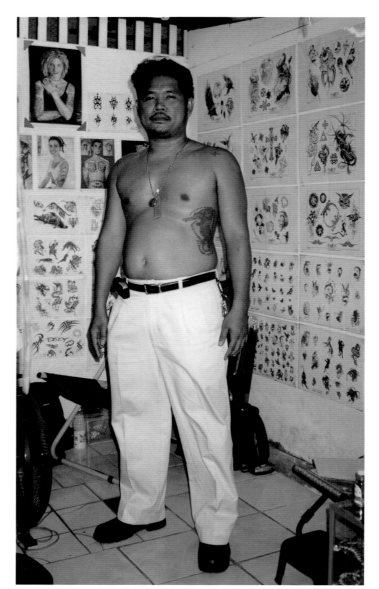

Pae in Ouy's booth.

Tattoos by Ouy

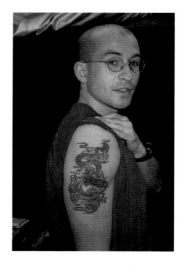
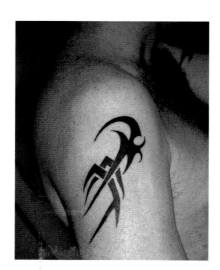
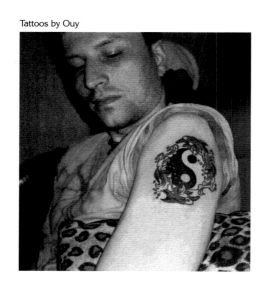

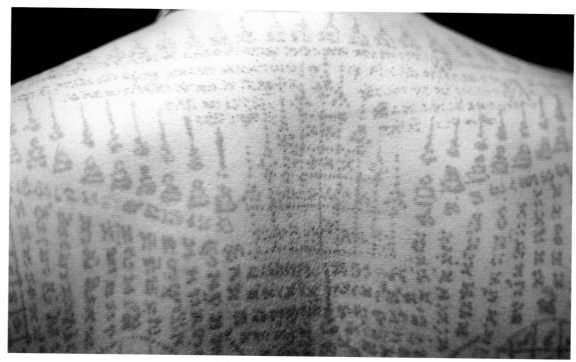

Pae's back tattooed with magical script.

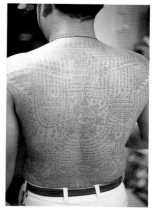

Pae's back tattooed with magical script.

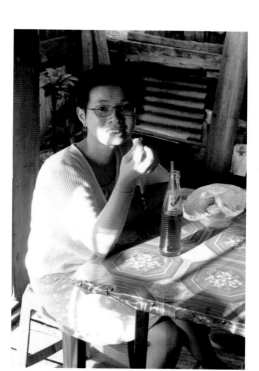

Lee

Indian Ruesi tattooed on Pae.

Pae chuckles respectfully as he looks at Ouy tattooing one of the Soi Cowboy girls with a small, generic western design on her lower back. "I see all these Thai people getting modern designs but it is not for me," he describes, gesturing towards the design. "I do not identify with these tattoos at all. I received my tattoos from monks. They blessed the image, the ink, and me. I made offerings to them out of respect for their power and skill. As they tattooed me they chanted spells meant to protect me and give me strength. When they finished, they touched me and blew on the fresh tattoo, which brought it to life."

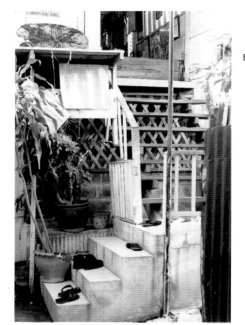

Entrance to Mr. Nue's studio.

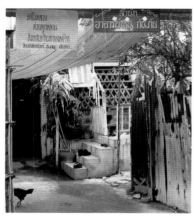

Entrance to Mr. Nue's studio.

In the outskirts of Bangkok, in the Pathumthanee district near the airport, a middle-aged tattoo magician named Mr. Nue has a reputation that extends throughout South East Asia for his powerful tattoos. He is known as a Black Magic Arjan. His studio is located at the end of a humble soi. Chickens scramble around the dirt road, chased by young kids and dogs with corkscrew tails. At the base of Mr. Nue's studio steps a few signs are tacked to the wall spelling his name in Thai. There are also three cow skulls with horns hanging on the wall that aren't necessarily menacing, they just hang there in the baking sun.

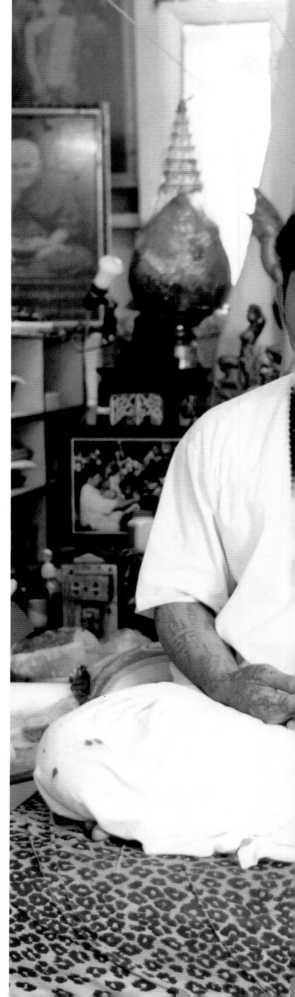

Mr. Nue.

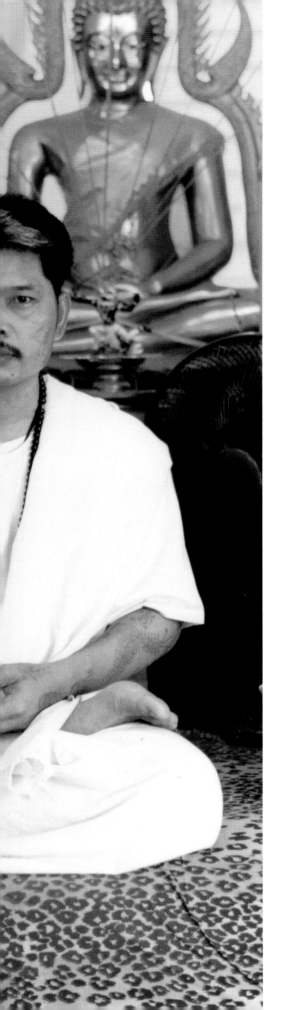

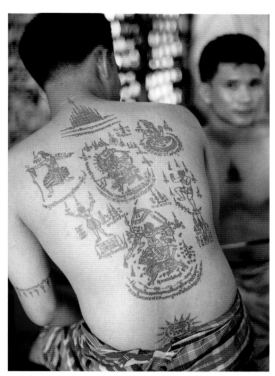

Magical charms by Mr. Nue.

"I see all these Thai people getting modern designs but it is not for me," I received my tattoos from monks. They blessed the image, the ink, and me. When they finished, they touched me and blew on the fresh tattoo, which brought it to life."

Upstairs, the Arjan's studio is large and airy, about 25-foot square with louvered windows at the back for cross ventilation. About 10 young men sit on the floor around two tattoo apprentices who are pushing ink with long traditional needle wands into two devotees. Mr. Nue sits in a meditative position surrounded by bowls and books. Some bowls have water in them, others have offerings of money from customers. To his left is a very crowded altar with several Buddhas. There are melted candles and incense sticks burning on the altar, and pieces of fabric with magical symbols that men fold up and wear. Along one wall of the studio glass display cases are full of esoteric artifacts: yellow candles with magical spells written into the wax, pieces of curled paper that have magical writing, small sculptures of animals.

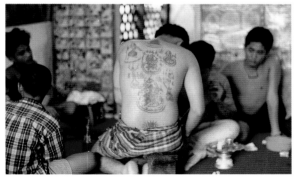

Interior Mr. Nue's studio.

13

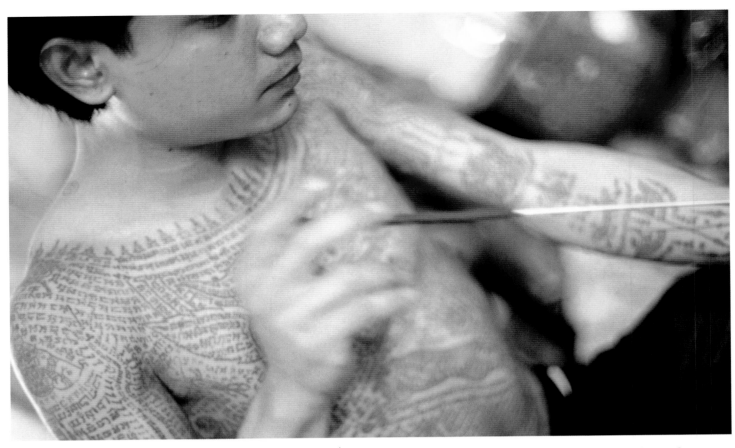

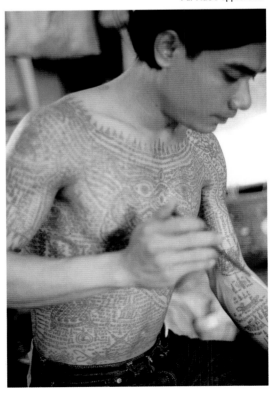

Mr. Nue's apprentice.

Mr. Nue used to be a Buddhist monk living for many years as a hermit deep in the jungle. He learned the secretive and sacred practice of conjuring tattoo magic from senior teachers when he was younger. His power is highly respected for the ability to change people's lives. He splits his time between his studio in Bangkok and a second shop in Malaysia.

He is not a median and does not claim to conjure spirits through himself. Rather, he knows the power of tattoos, and applies them onto customers so they can heal or change themselves. It is the person wearing the tattoo who is powerful. The tattoo helps them to find the power in themselves.

Two younger students are working at the Arjan's feet tattooing sacred images onto customers. They are both heavily tattooed from the neck to the belt level with Khmer language script. Nestled into the script are images of Hindu deities, Shiva, Brahma, Vishnu, and Ganesha. There are Buddhist deities as well. These images first made their way to Indochina around 500 A.D. from China and India following old trade routes. They were adopted by ancient Khmer people and synthesized into a fluid belief system that incorporated them with traditional local animist beliefs. People spun them all together to help control the unpredictable nature of their lives. One of Mr. Nue's patrons has his entire back tattooed with an Avatar turtle image that is made from Khmer script. The Avatar played a key role in Khmer iconography, being associated with longevity and the ancient Khmer creation myth of The Churning of the Milk.

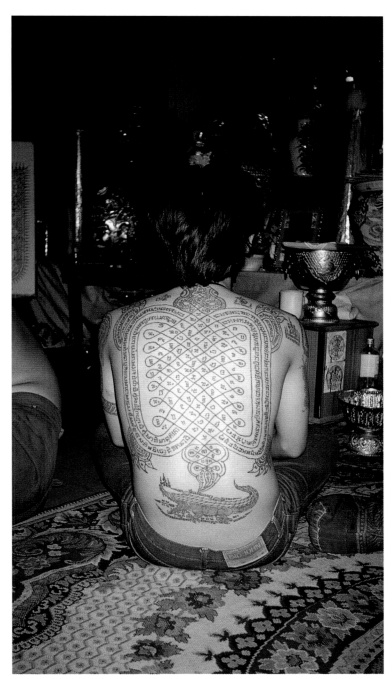

Magical Avatar tattoo by Mr. Nue.

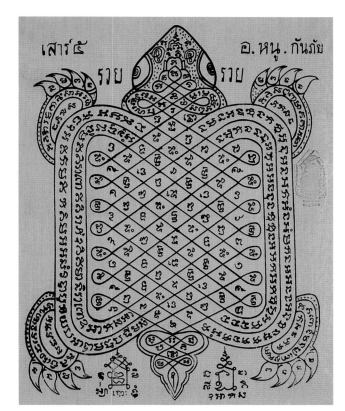

Magical spirit cloth of Avatar image.

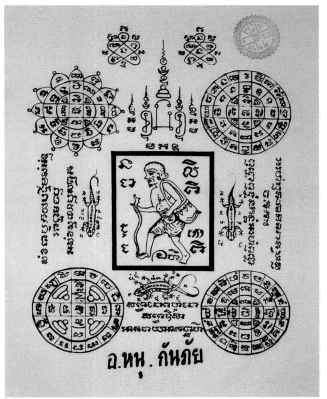

Spirit cloth with Indian Ruesi hermit.

The Khmer script Mr. Nue has tattooed onto his apprentices has been done in a mysterious fashion. He explains through a translator, "Changes have been made in the Khmer verse that prevents people from reading it. Letters have been jumbled or left out, words have been abbreviated; parts of designs like a tiger's tail have been eliminated or changed to lessen the power. I know the secret code I have worked into the tattooed spells. I guard it carefully to prevent the possibility of powerful counter-magic. Some designs are so powerful, I change them to prevent the wearer from going insane."

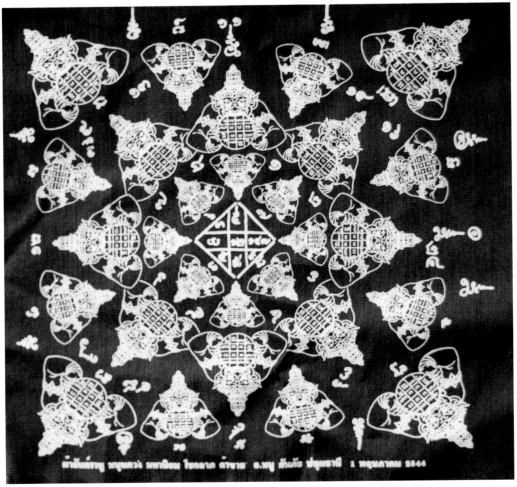

Magical spirit cloth at Mr. Nue's studio for strength.

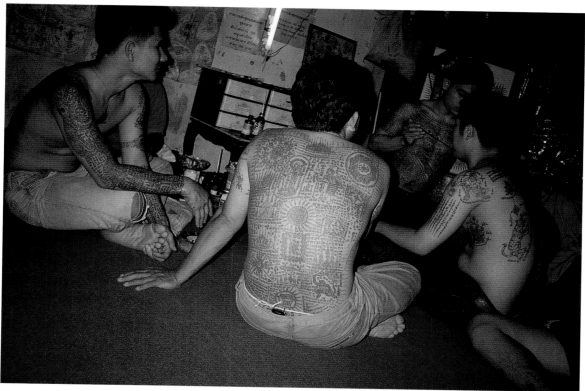

Tattoos by Mr. Nue's apprentice.

Tattoos by Mr. Nue's apprentice.

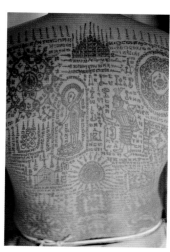

Tattoo by Mr. Nue. Note image of Ganesh.

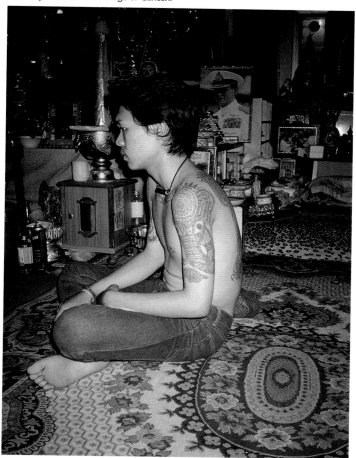

Tattoo by Mr. Nue's apprentice. Note image of Hanuman (bottom) and Vishnu (left).

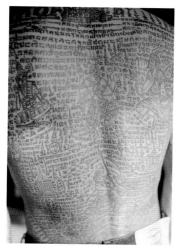

The tattoos on the apprentices have a power point called the *heart*. During the tattooing process, Mr. Nue has recited sacred syllables or a mantra at the same time he puts power into the heart. Without reciting the mantra, the tattooed letters have no power. The heart is placed at the beginning, middle, or end of the tattooed design or script. The person wearing the tattoo does not know the location of the heart. Anyone with this information can make the tattoo powerless.

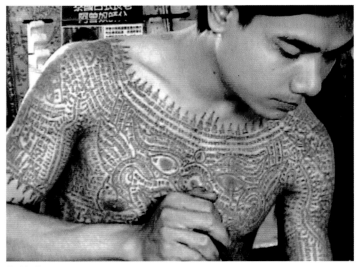

Mr. Nue's apprentice tattooing.

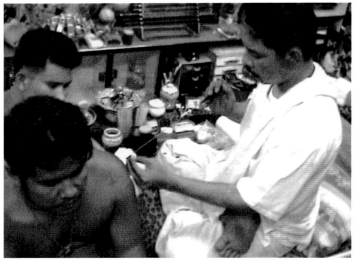

Mr. Nue tattooing.

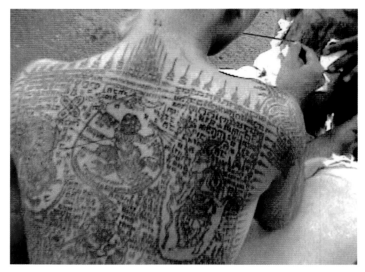

Mr. Nue's second apprentice tattooing.

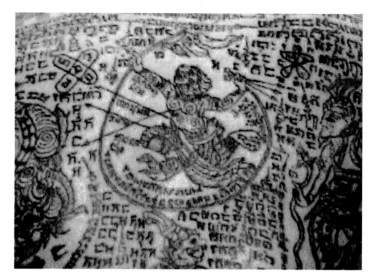
Tattoos on Mr. Nue's second apprentice.

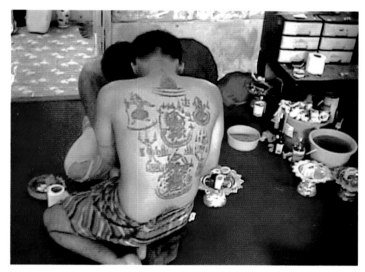
Tattoo devotee at Mr. Nue's Studio

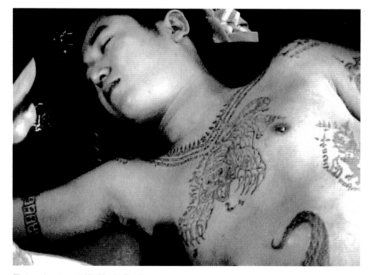
Tattoo devotee at Mr. Nue's Studio

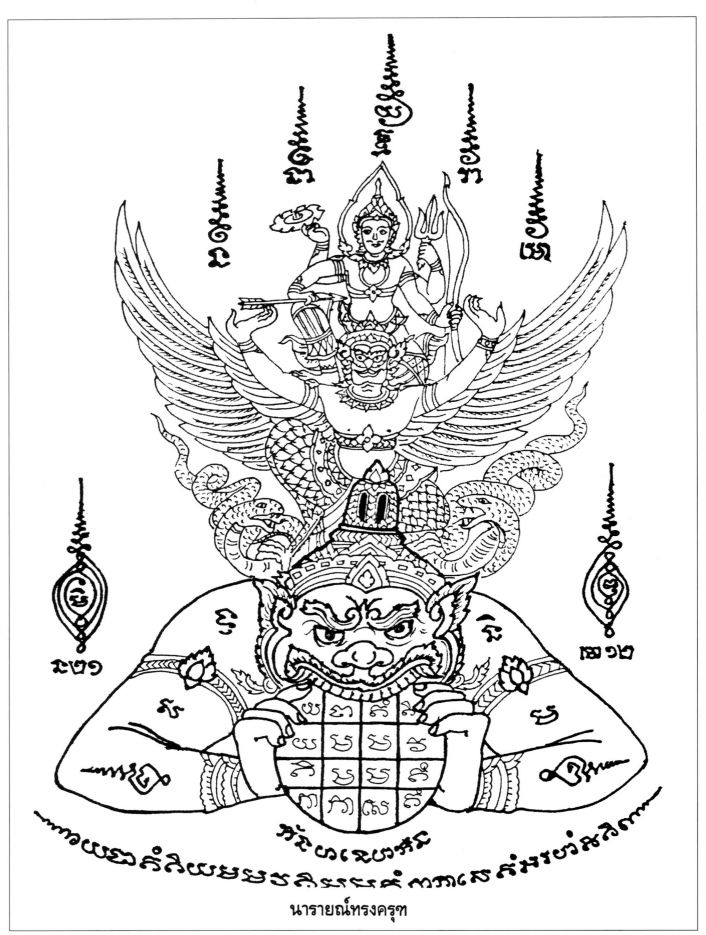

นารายณ์ทรงครุฑ

Vishnu riding Garuda, Mr. Nue's studio.

As the arjan, Mr. Nue monitors the progress of the tattoos being applied by his apprentices. When they are completed, the customers approach him for a blessing. As they kneel in front of him, he incants some phrases, wipes at the fresh blood with his fingers and then blows forcefully on the new tattoo. The customers bow forward respectfully, their hands at their nose.

It is very rare for a woman to be tattooed this way. Mr. Nue has tattooed a young lady who is a Bangkok performing celebrity, but it is extremely rare. Traditional tattooing in Indochina is the domain of men. Women are thought to drain the power of the tattoos, a prohibition associated with the monthly cycle of menstruation. The loss of blood is thought to drain the power of the Arjan and tattoo; association with it is avoided.

Mr. Nue and his apprentices represent the bridge between the traditional tattoo practices in countries like Thailand, Cambodia, Laos, Burma, and Vietnam, and the infusion of modern, western imagery and motivations that is accelerating very quickly in the region. Men, young and old, continue to patronize Mr. Nue, hoping they can use his guidance and skill to improve their lives.

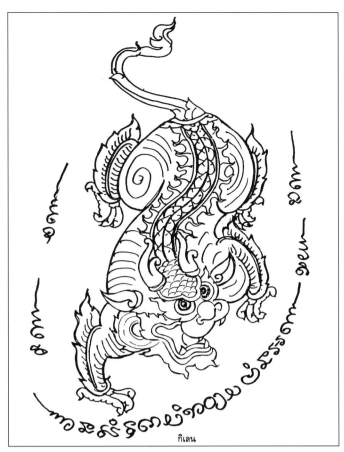

Khmer lion design from Mr. Nue's studio.

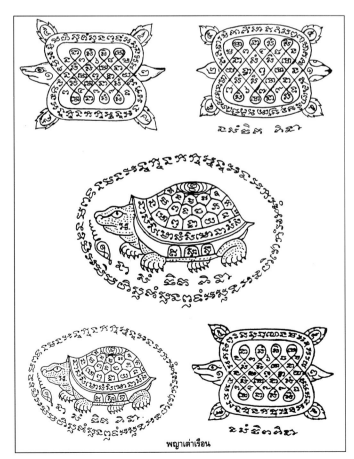

Avatar images from Mr. Nue's studio.

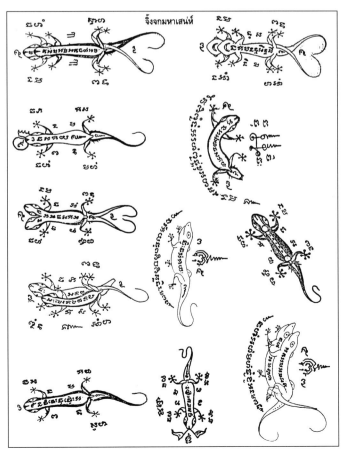

Jing-Jok designs from Mr. Nue's studio.

21

Chapter Two

BANGKOK TATTOO

The streets of Bangkok, Thailand, are a danger-ous whir of relentless chaos. Small motorcycles with sexy women riding sidesaddle spin fearlessly through the maze of constantly gridlocked trucks and econo-sized cars. Pedestrians run for their lives, gauging safe tolerances between tank-like homicidal busses and runaway, three-wheeled Tuk-Tuk taxis. Saffron robed Buddhist monks glide through it all as if they are float-ing. Their shoulders are tattooed with elaborate pro-tective amulets and sacred script. Passersby dip their heads in respect as they cross the monk's path. Dazed opium addicts are secreted away in dark, neglected corners between buildings. They stare into space as if they are dead.

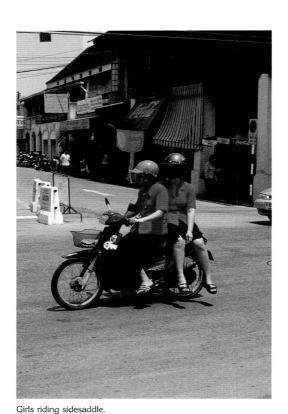

Girls riding sidesaddle.

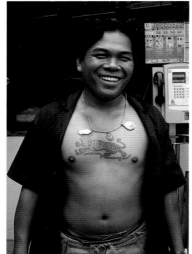

Bangkok Tuk-Tuk driver with tiger tattoo.

Bangkok alleyway.

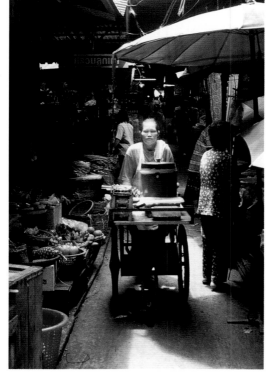

Bangkok Tuk-Tuk driver.

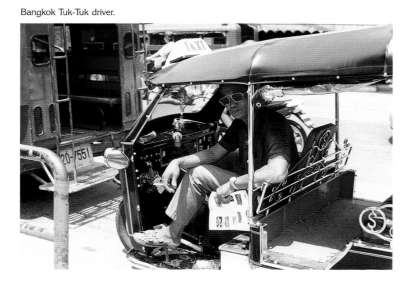

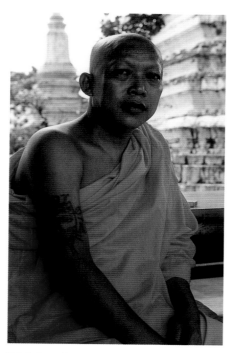

Bangkok monk.

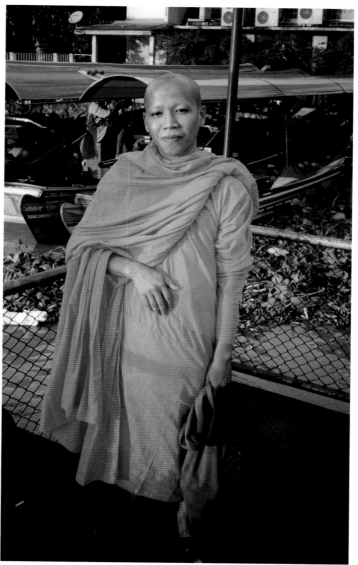

Bangkok monk.

Opium addict tattooing Bangkok club girl.

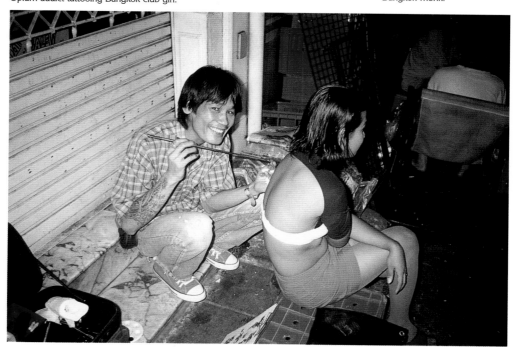

Tattoo graffiti in Bangkok alley.

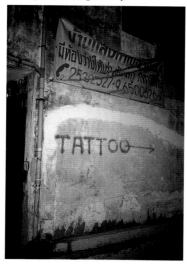

At night the city shifts into an exotic overdrive. There are few streetlights and the darkness seems thick and mysterious. Sidewalk peddlers are illuminated briefly by the sweep of passing car headlights; their mannerisms and facial expressions become chopped up in stroboscopic abbreviation as money changes hands. On some streets, elephants appear magically from alleyways. Tethered by their keepers, the huge animals dance through the traffic, led to some illegal work. Elephants have been banned in the city for years but they remain.

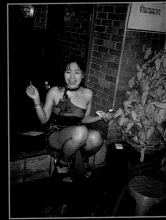

Bangkok club girl.

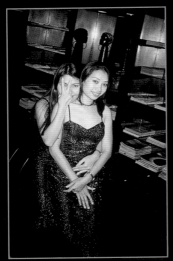

Bangkok club girls.

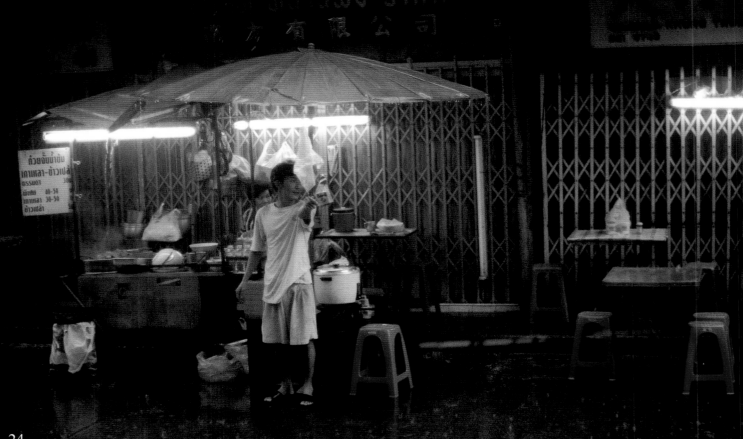

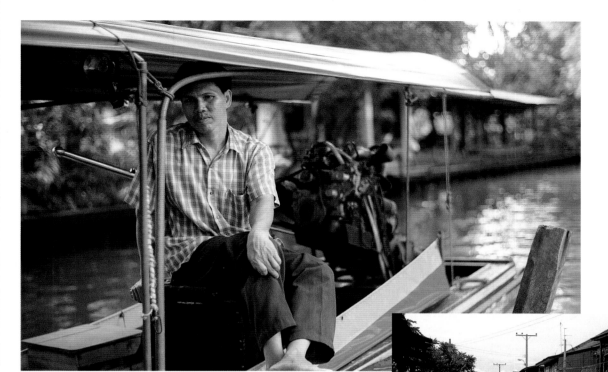

Bangkok water taxi driver.

Bangkok sidewalk.

Bangkok klong.

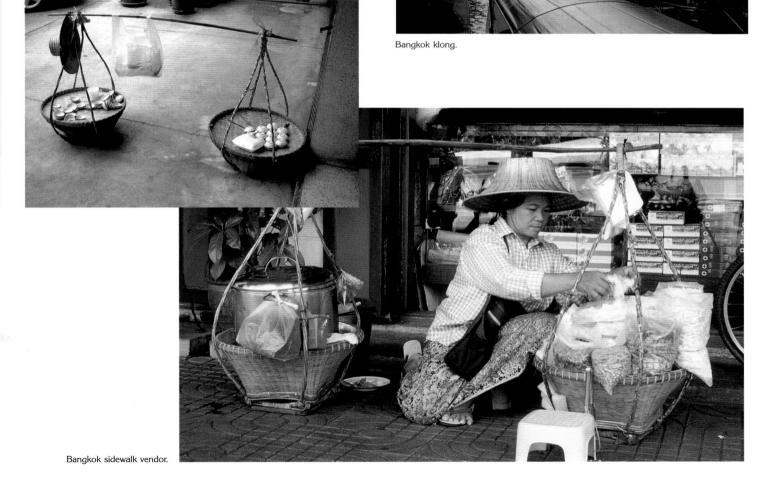

Bangkok sidewalk vendor.

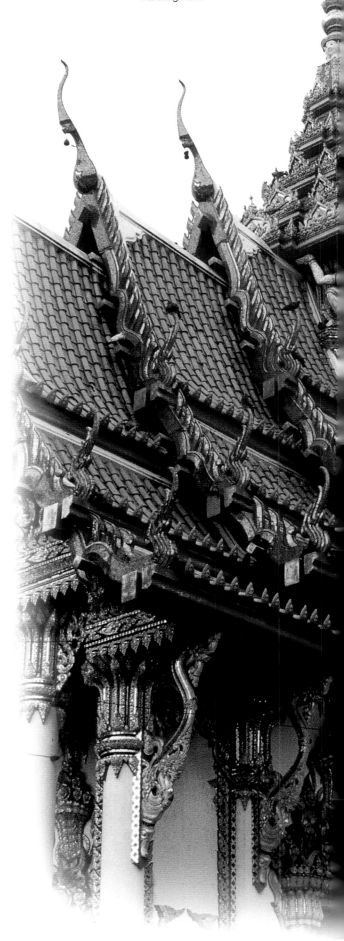

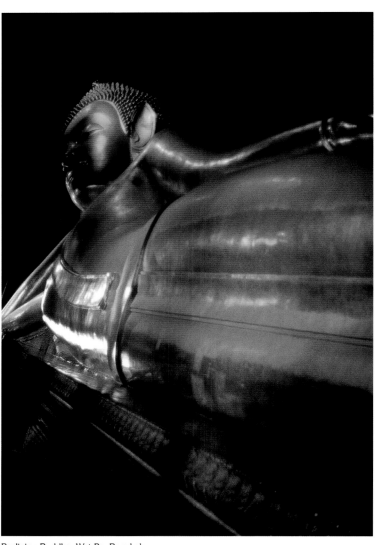

Reclining Buddha, Wat Po, Bangkok.

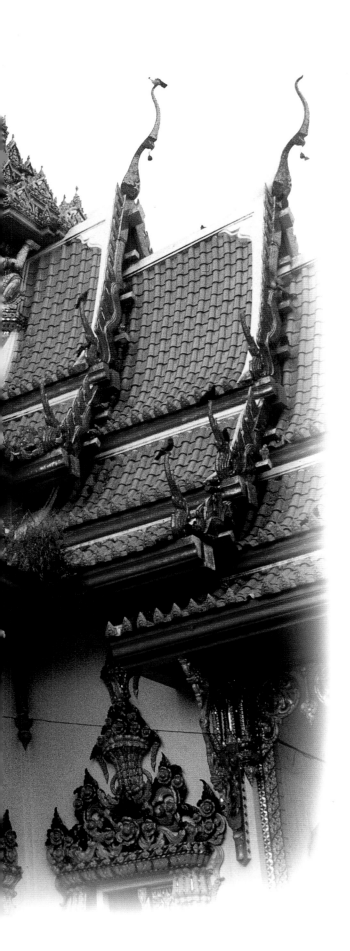

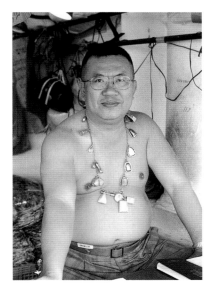

Man wearing magical amulets.

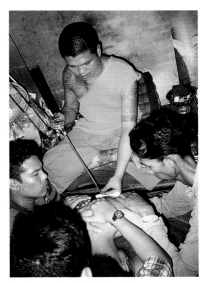

Monk tattooing at Wat Bang Phraw.

Young Thai girls in their twenties cluster in front of the classy hostess clubs along Sukhumvit Road. They sit on the club steps, bobbing one leg off their knee, smoking cigarettes. Like schools of flowing fish, they spill into the street in coordinated eveningwear outfits flashing toothy smiles, grabbing at the arms of passing male pedestrians, coaxing them into the clubs. There are dozens of bars back-to-back down the street with names like Luciano's and Club Renior. Nightlife gets dangerous in the Pat Pong district and on Soi Nana and Soi Cowboy. The girls there become carnivorous, lunging first at zippers and then unprotected wallets. Drunk European men slap feebly at the swarm of delicate piranha hands.

Tattoos infiltrate the entire culture in Bangkok. Traditional Buddhist protective charms peek from behind older men's shirt collars and waistbands. The images have been used for hundreds of years for physical and spiritual strength and persevere as potent symbols. Many men have been tattooed at the temple called, Wat Bang Phraw, which is located 40 kilometers Northwest of Bangkok in the Nakhon Chaisri province. The monks there are known for tattooing the image of a pouncing tiger on the chest. The master monk has a reputation for riding wild tigers after he has calmed them with his meditative power and young devotees fuse with this power through their tattoos.

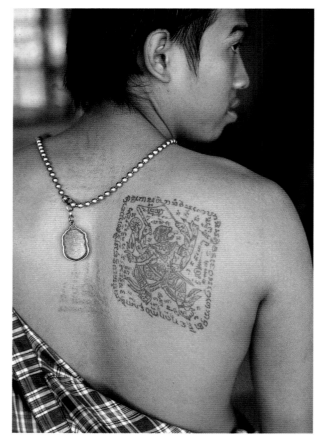

Patron at Wat Bang Phraw

Patrons at Wat Bang Phraw.

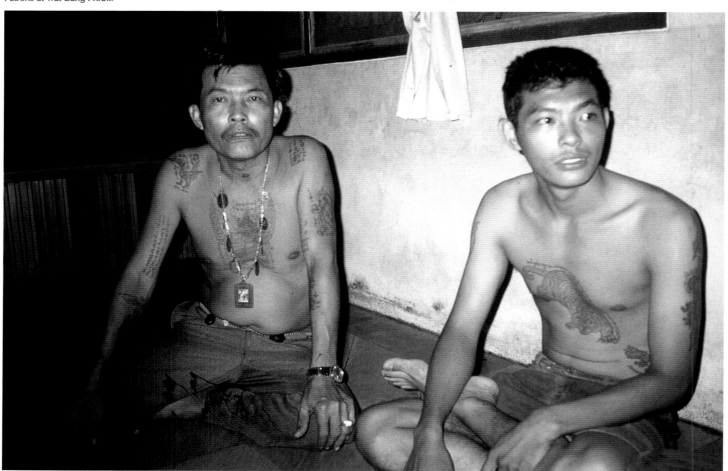

The tattoo charms serve a variety of purposes that are both sacred and secular. Some help to find a wife or make money. Others make the wearer bulletproof or uncuttable with knives. Many times the tattoos are applied with anointed oil rather than ink. The images become nearly invisible but are just as powerful.

Magical tattoos, Wat Bang Phraw

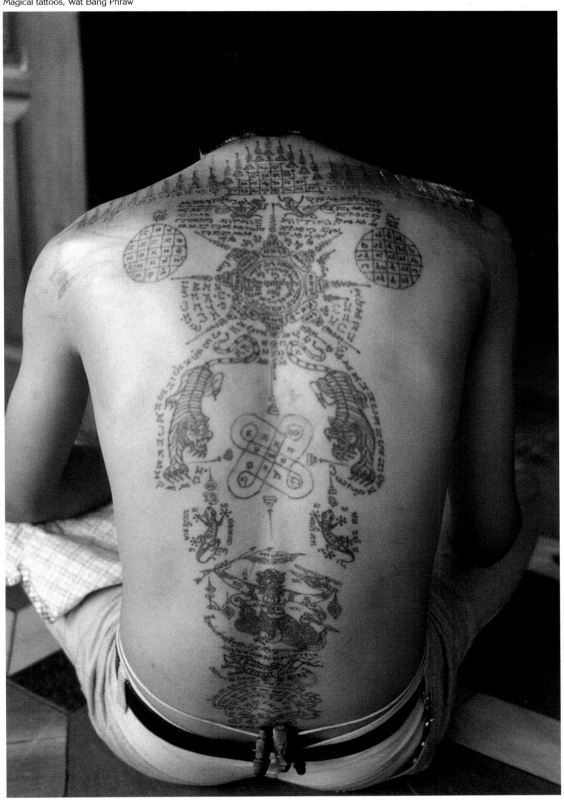

In contrast, on Bangkok streets and in nightclubs some urban teens flaunt Pop tattoo images that connect them to a distant Western world. In a reversed flow, Bangkok youth grab at the exotic allure of American brand name, everything from Nike sneakers to tattoo iconography. Wearing a Western-style tattoo projects a connection to the future at the same time that it tacitly reinforces the Thai tattoo tradition. The images have changed, but the motivations to be marked with powerful amulets may be the same. For many Thai urban youth, the Nike logo or obvious western style tattoos represent power. No heads turn in surprise to any of it; tattoos of some kind have been a part of Thai life since at least 500 A.D. and Khmer times and it all seems to have a natural place.

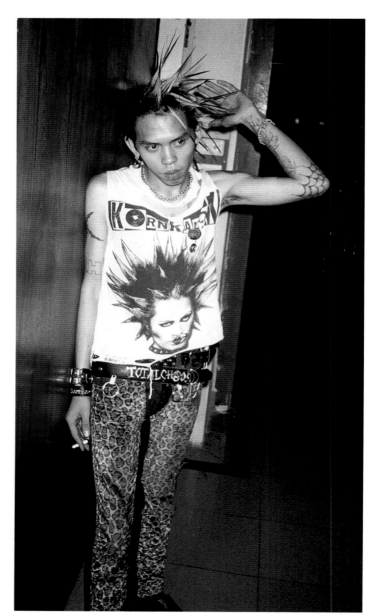

Tattooed youth at Bangkok nightclub.

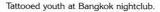

Tattooed youth at Bangkok nightclub.

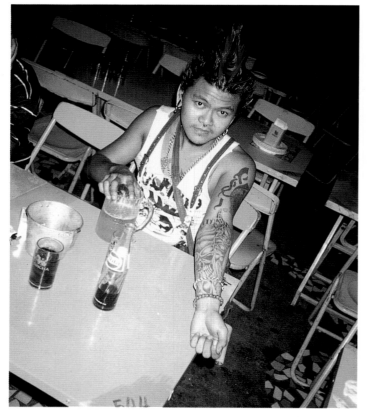

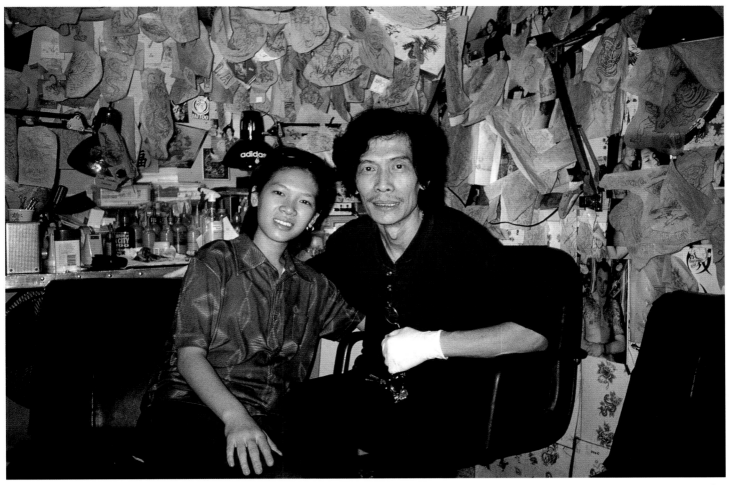

Jimmy Wong with his daughter Joy.

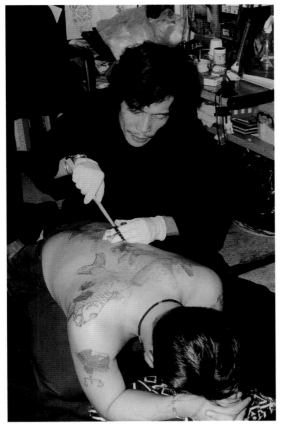

Jimmy Wong tattooing with hand tools.

Jimmy Wong has been tattooing in Bangkok since the 1970s and the Vietnam War period. He now has three shops located in different parts of the city. His daughter Joy works from one on the first floor of the Mahboonkron Shopping Center. His son Jukkoo works at another located at Soi 35/60, Wattanawong Makkasan, and Jimmy works next to the Fortuna Hotel on Sukhumvit Road, Soi 5. "I started my tattooing at the end of the Vietnam War," he explains. "I tattooed a lot of American GIs. I worked up on the Thai-Laos boarder. There was an American airbase there. Every payday I was very busy. Not so many GIs came down to Bangkok. It was too far away. I tattooed 'Mom and Dad', eagles and anchors on the Navy guys. It was all military style. After the war, I came back to Bangkok."

31

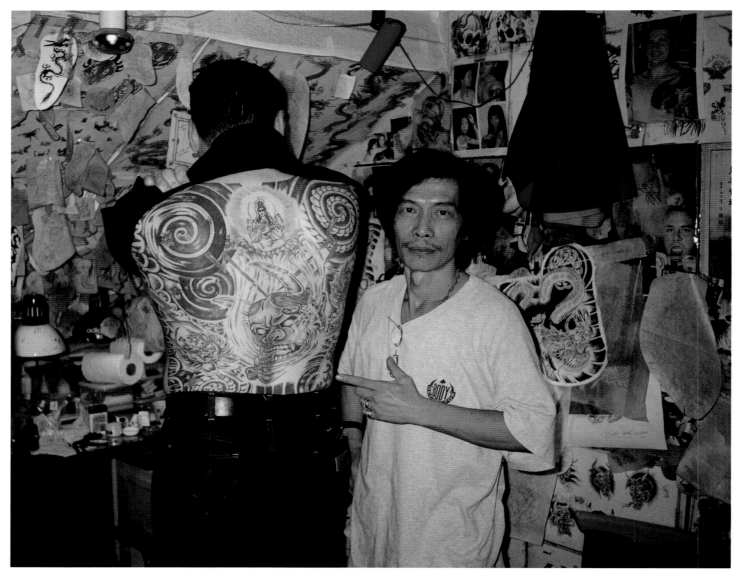

Jimmy Wong

Tattoo by Jimmy Wong.

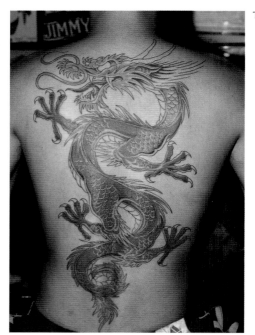

"In my country they have two kinds of tattooing now. One is traditional, from monks and tattoo masters. The master decides how to design a tattoo. He uses elements to create the design for good luck and protect yourself so nobody can hurt you, protect your vision, good business; if you need a wife… Western style tattooing came in not so long ago. The 'art style' tattoos started with the GIs but they've really only been popular for 15 years."

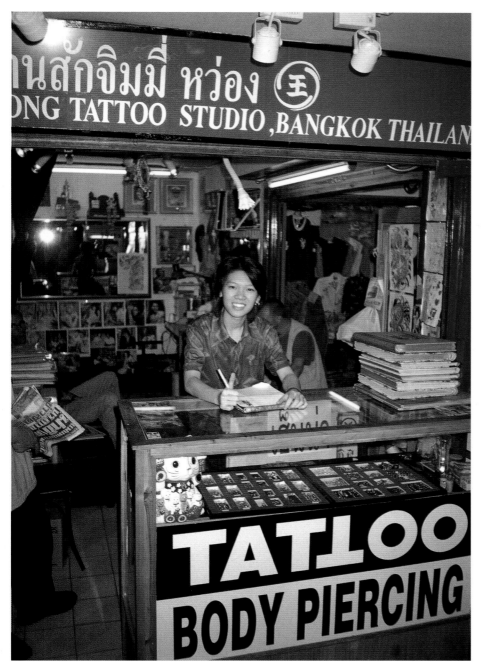

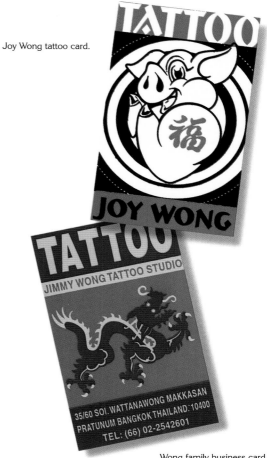

Joy Wong at her tattoo shop.

Joy Wong tattoo card.

Wong family business card.

Joy Wong Tattooing.

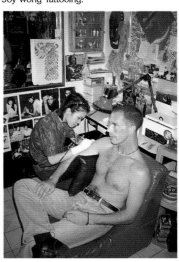

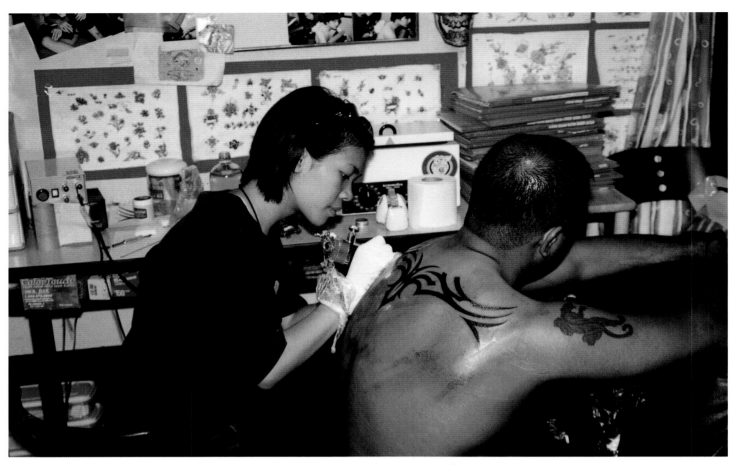

Joy Wong tattooing.

Hanuman tattoo by Jimmy Wong

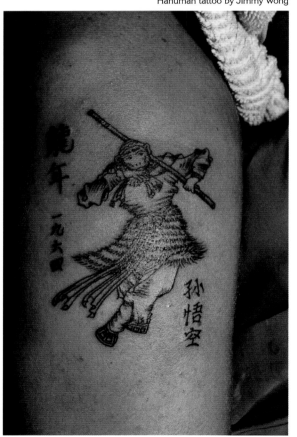

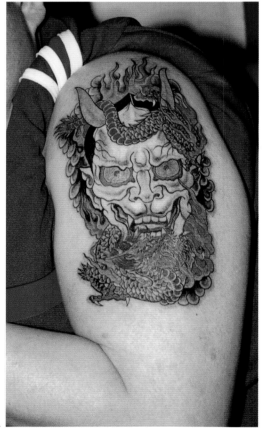

Tattoo by Joy Wong.

"In my country they have two kinds of tattooing now. One is traditional, from monks and tattoo masters. The master decides how to design a tattoo. He uses elements to create the design for good luck and protect yourself so nobody can hurt you, protect your vision, good business; if you need a wife… Western style tattooing came in not so long ago. The 'art style' tattoos started with the GIs but they've really only been popular for 15 years. Thai people have been following the styles of many magazines and movie stars.

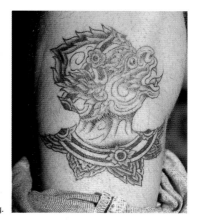

Tattoo by Jimmy Wong.

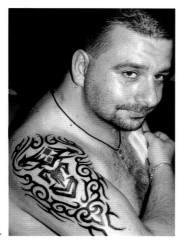

Tattoo by Joy Wong.

Tattoo by Joy Wong.

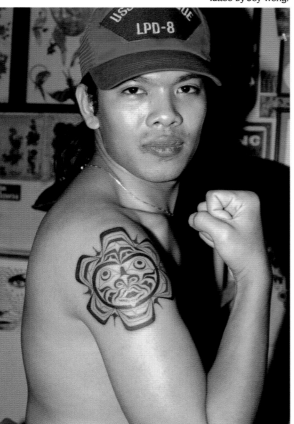

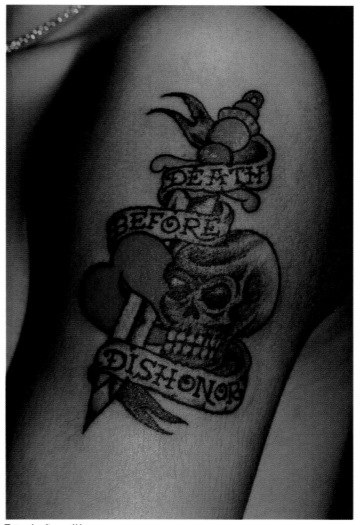

Tattoo by Jimmy Wong

"The world is changing now. There is more contact. Magazines and TV shows- people follow the fashion. I still keep my old style: Thai and Asian style. In my country the tattoo styles are a part of the culture. Good meaning of the tattoos, not cartoons or new style work. We don't understand those images. In my shop, many people come for traditional styles that have traditional meanings — like the dragon. We do many dragons because that is a special animal for us. We've had these images for a long time in Asia.

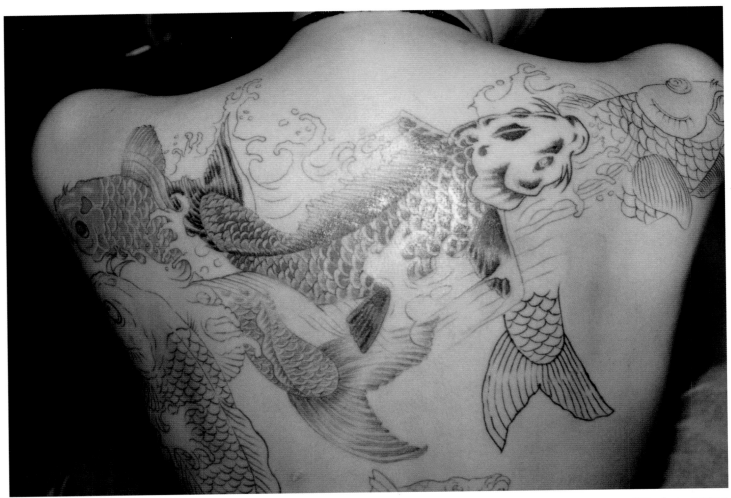

Tattoo by Jimmy Wong.

"I think that tattoo artists are the same everywhere. We all put ink into the skin. We are connected in that way no matter where we tattoo. I think that the meanings of the tattoos are different. What we all design shows our feelings and our different cultures. That is the difference between us. I have been in Europe and America and Japan. Tattooers are no different in any of these places. We are all the same when we use the ink.

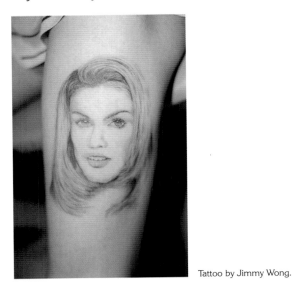

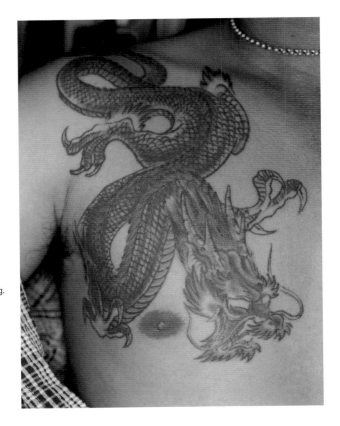

Tattoo by Jimmy Wong.

Tattoo by Jimmy Wong.

36

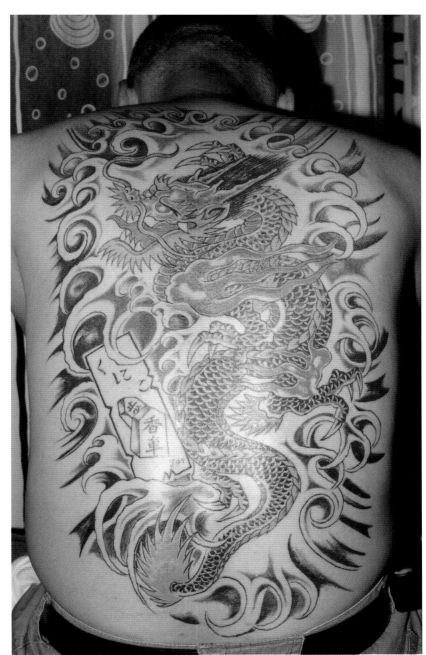

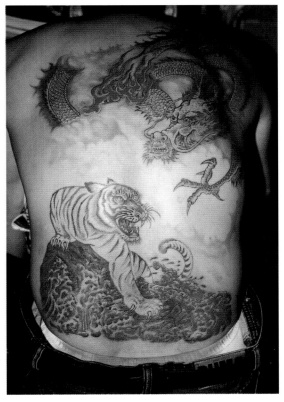

"Today many people follow the fashion to get tattooed. For me, this is not good. I don't advertise my shop. People that come here already know what they are doing. They know what they want. I just don't tattoo anybody. I have to know that the person is doing the right thing. I think like the Buddha says — you have to do something good. I want to do good things and get a good thing back. Thailand is a Buddhist country. I think about this kind of thing. I want to do the good thing for people, then you get back the good thing. I listen to the Buddhist path — how to use my life to do good."

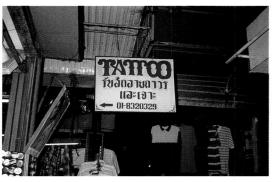

Tattoo sign, Ja-Too-Jak market.

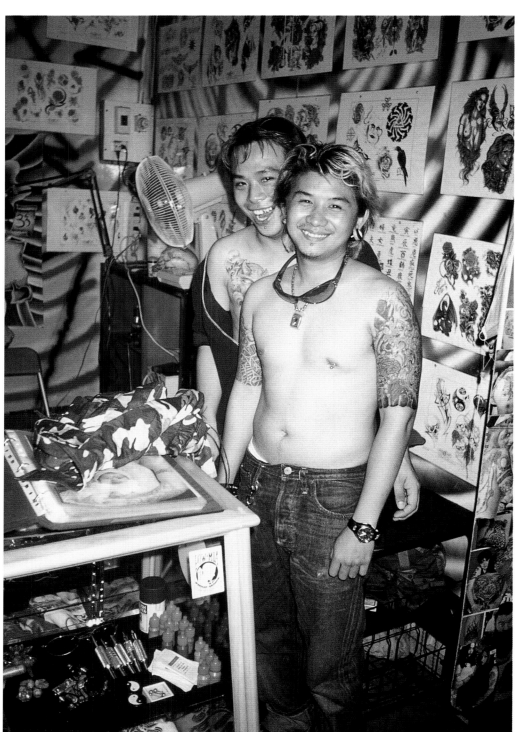

Young tattoo enthusiasts at Ja-Too-Jak market.

Unlike Jimmy, most Bangkok tattooers are new to the trade. They have jumped on the global bandwagon of popularity and only recently established shops in places like the Ja-Too-Jak weekend market, located in the northwestern section of the city. The covered market area is a dizzying honeycomb of passageways, crammed with small shops selling everything from kitchenware to food, clothing, jewelry, and pirated audio CDs. At every turn there is a cramped booth with a hand-painted sign out front advertising tattooing. Some are simple with little fanfare: Just a single tattooer working humbly — maybe a girlfriend smoking a cigarette quietly in the background. Others have display counters full of nondescript tattoo machines and piercing jewelry, and a boom box blaring American, Rock and Roll. In these more elaborate booths, there are enlarged photos of western tattooed people tacked to the wall and piles of battered tattoo magazines from Europe and the USA. The preoccupation with western culture is acute here.

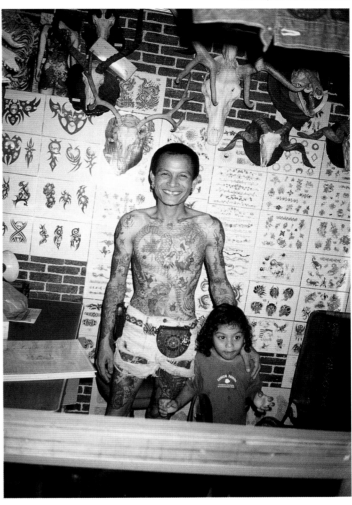

Tattooer, Ja-Too-Jak market.

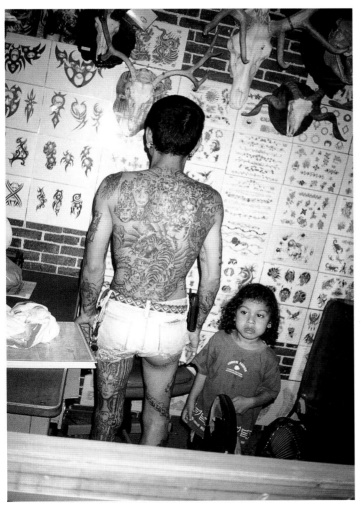

Tattooer, Ja-Too-Jak market.

" I think like the Buddha says — you have to do something good. I want to do good things and get a good thing back. Thailand is a Buddhist country. I think about this kind of thing. I want to do the good thing for people, then you get back the good thing. I listen to the Buddhist path — how to use my life to do good."

39

The customers are mostly males in their late teens and early twenties. Many have trendy, dyed hair and wear hip T-shirts. They turn the pages of the portfolios hoping to connect to an image. Few if any have traditional Thai tattooed charms, but most wear Buddhist amulet necklaces. Something is both in and out of sync between their hunger for generic Western tattoo designs and the richness of this culture. A reflection of the ambiguity of our times. One young tattooer named Puy has a loose-leaf notebook in his booth full of traditional Buddhist charm designs he has collected. "These tattoos are very old," he reflects in labored, broken English. "Young people don't look at them much now. They look better at the pictures from America. They want the pictures from America. I keep these for a few people who want them. Not too many any more in Bangkok, everything America now…"

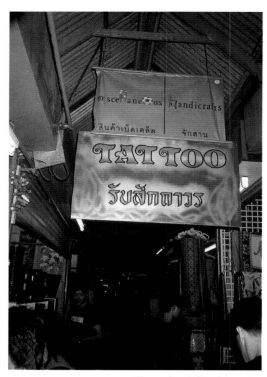

Tattoo sign, Ja-Too-Jak market.

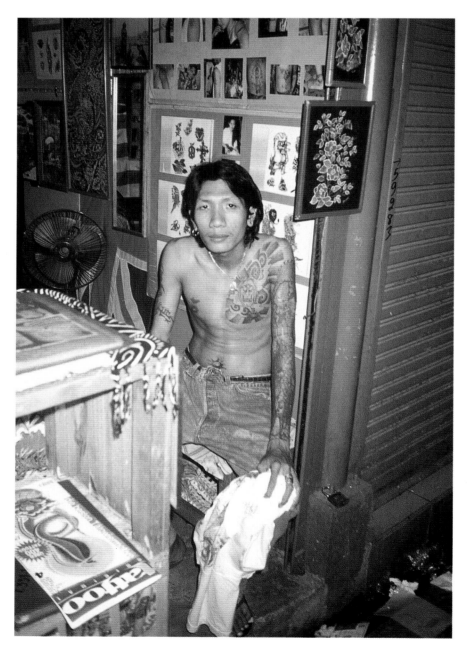

Tattoo enthusiast, Ja-Too-Jak market.

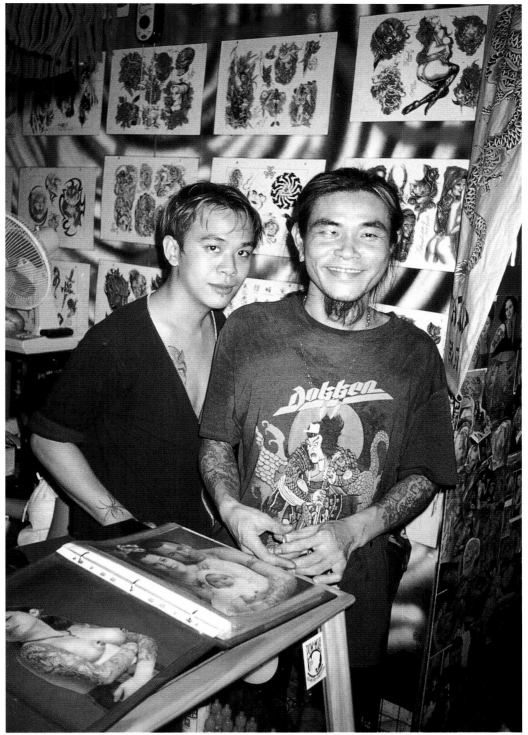

Tattoo artist, Ja-Too-Jak market.

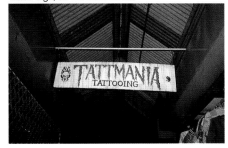

Tattoo Sign, Ja-Too-Jak market.

It is hard to predict what will happen with tattooing in a place like Bangkok. Traditional images and motivations are fading among the younger generation as they surrender to the West. The infatuation is confused at the same time that it is intense. Global substitutes continue to erode distinct, traditional tattoo practices that have flourished for thousands of years. Possibly some hybrid combination will develop between the sacred and profane that serves to bridge the two.

41

Chapter Three

TESTING THE SPELL

THE TATTOOS AT
WAT LAN DONG

Heads turn as we pull into the dusty temple grounds of Wat Lan Dong. Two young men standing 25 feet off the ground on thrown together scaffolding smile as they look down at us from under their wide-brimmed straw hats. They hammer away at sun bleached wooden molding, knocking it off the steep roofline of the humble, sacred structure that looks hundreds of years old. The exotic, flame-shaped detailing had once been a rich, deep red with gold edging, but the intensity is gone.

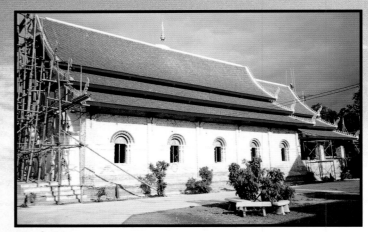

Wat Lan Dong

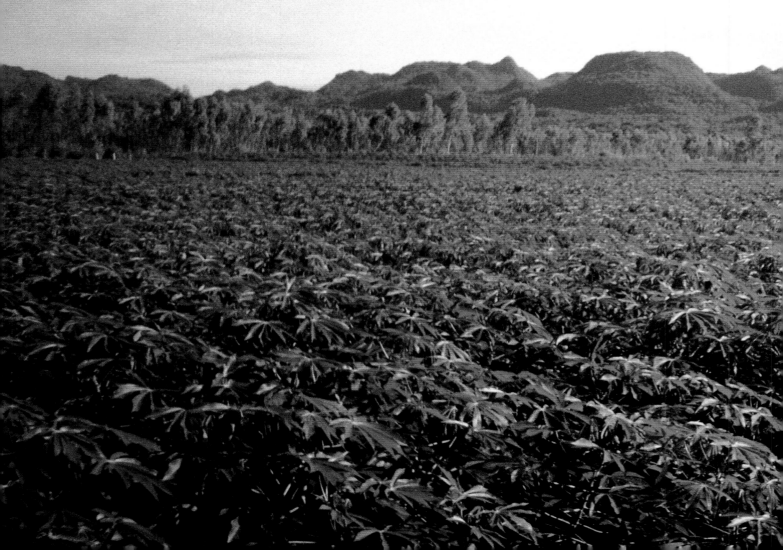

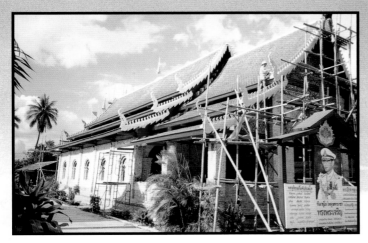

Wat Lan Dong

Three young novice monks wearing saffron robes stir from inside the temple as my driver parks his Tuk-Tuk under a shade tree. They walk towards us into the bright sun with a shielding hand cupped at their brow. Underfed dogs prance along next to them, sniffing the scent of strangers.

The 40 Kilometer drive from Chiang Mai had taken us north along a two-lane paved road through manicured agricultural areas backed up against steep, forest-green mountains. My driver Sammy has a brother living in the area who received traditional, magical tattoos from the young monk at the temple. He is on his way to meet us and arrange for the monk to do a large tiger tattoo meant to protect Sammy from the slice of a knife.

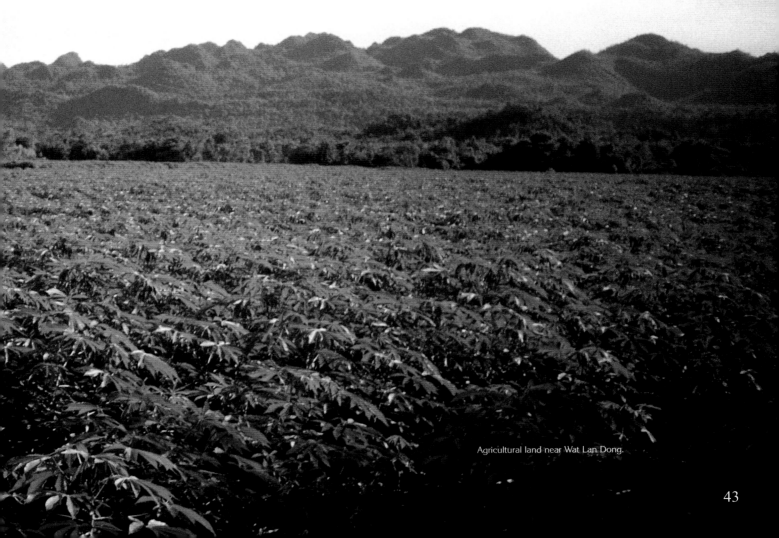

Agricultural land near Wat Lan Dong.

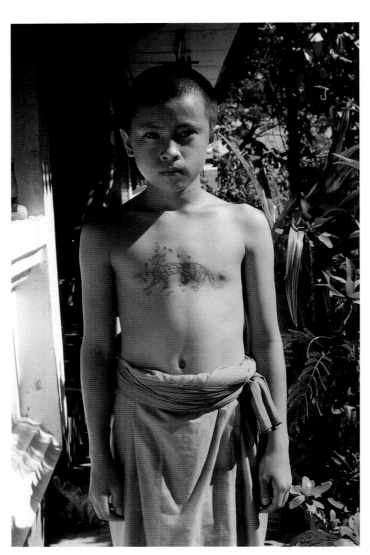

The youngest of the three novices looks to be around 12 years old. The bristles of his short-cropped black hair glisten in the intense sunlight. The robe he wears partially covers his youthful chest and the tiger design he has tattooed across it. We follow as he leads us through the dusty temple grounds towards a long garage-like building where the tattoo monk Tischa Padoom is sitting cross-legged on a red carpet. He is young and looks surprised to see us standing at the doorway. The room is sparsely furnished; a chair, a short table, and some boxes that are stacked up in the corners. Young men are enthusiastically watching a color television set that is tuned to a program of kickboxing. They nod their heads as we move through the room before they return to the boxing. Two middle-aged men are at the monk's feet, bowing respectfully and placing offerings in a metal bowl. A second bowl with tooled designs on it is full of water. The monk dips his fingers into the water and shakes them over the men's heads while reciting spells. Each of the bowing men has several tattoos on their chest, arms, and thighs of sacred Khmer script and Buddhist and Hindu deities. One of the men has a large tumorous lump on his forehead that is completely tattooed with a magical, spiral-like design. He turns momentarily towards us, squinting.

12-year-old novice monk with tiger chest tattoo.

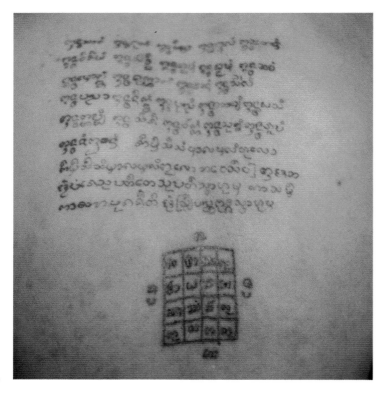

Sacred back tattoo on temple devotee.

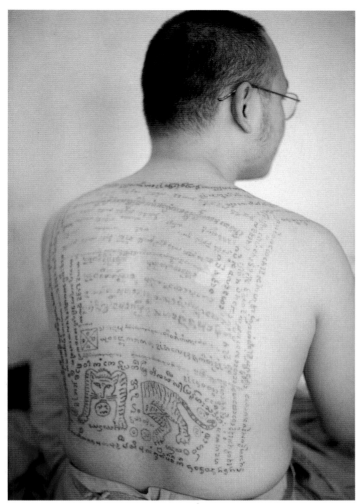

Monk Tischa Padoom's back tattoos.

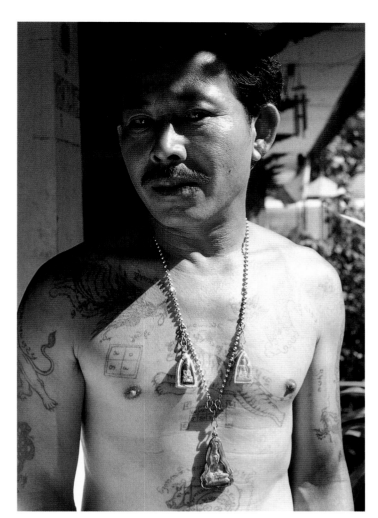

Sammy's brother

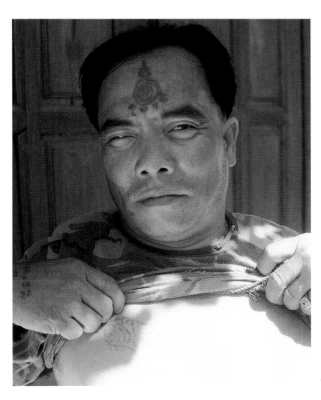

Temple devotee with tattooed tumor.

"There are hundreds of small temples like this throughout Thailand where monks do magical tattooing," Sammy describes. "Some have developed wide reputations while others are known only to the people that live near them. The temples survive from the offerings people make for the tattoos."

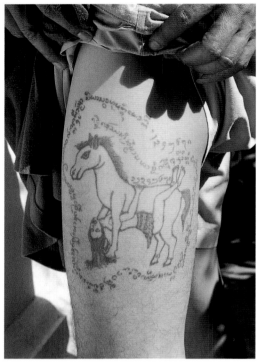

Leg tattoo on Sammy's brother meant to enhance sexual power. Tattoos below the waist are usually sexual in nature.

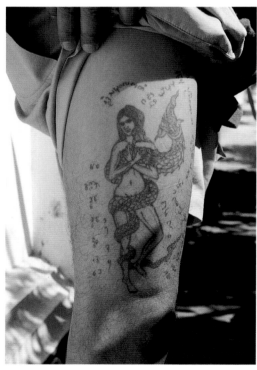

Leg tattoo on Sammy's brother meant to enhance sexual power.

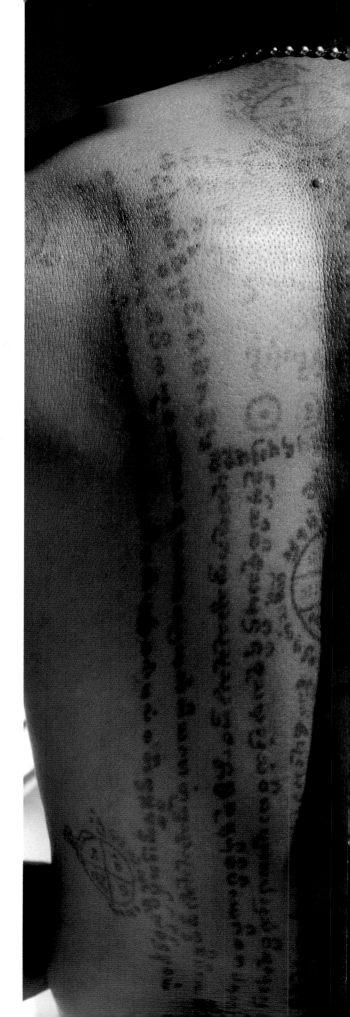

46

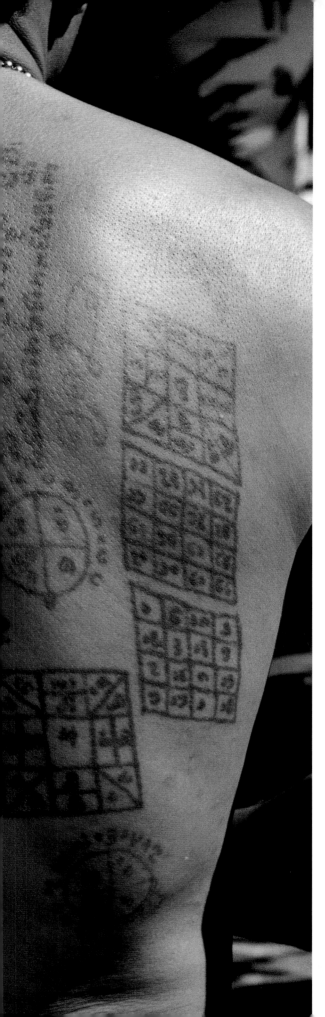

Yantric astrological tattoos on Sammy's brother's back.

There are temples in all the countries of Indochina where magical tattooing continues to be practiced although most believe that enthusiasm for tattooing is greatest in Thailand. The popularity of magical tattooing confuses some people and is associated with gangsterism and the life of the underworld. Bowing to social pressure, sesame oil is sometimes used instead of ink to create nearly invisible tattooed charms.

Temple devotee tattooed with sacred phrases, Yantra and animal images.

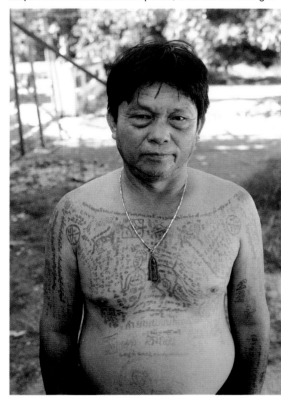

Sammy's brother arrives and talks with the monk about the tiger tattoo. The monk waves my driver over to his side and motions for the young novice with the tiger chest tattoo to gather some needles. The boy takes a few over to a common household hotplate, rests them onto the heating element and turns it on. As the needles heat up and turn a gentle red, the monk fingers through a long, thin book with hand lettering in it. He pauses occasionally, studying specific pages then flips past as if he is looking for a phone number. Finally, he settles into the text on one page, lifts the book, and bends the spine back to keep his place. There is a second book full of designs: strange images of human-like forms that look like they are floating in space surrounded with Khmer text. Sammy sees the image and explains, "This image is a powerful charm meant to prevent drowning. The pictures in the monk's book have been passed down to him. Men have used magical tattoos to ensure their safety for a long time. When a man would leave a village, he would protect himself against jungle spirits, bandits, and wild animals."

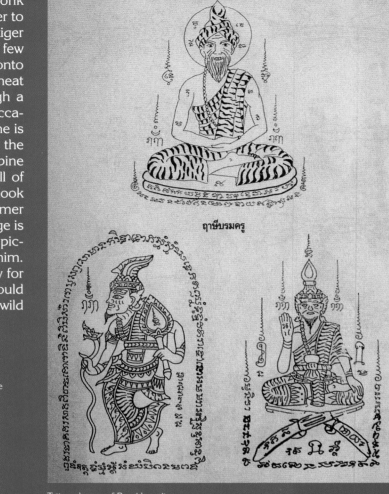

ฤๅษีบรมครู

Tattoo charms of Ruesi hermit.

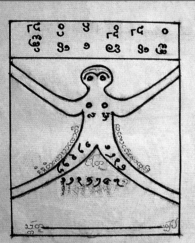

Magical tattoo charm image to prevent drowning.

Other pages have designs comprised of groups of Brahmanical Yantric squares or Yan with magical Khmer lettering. These Yantric designs are sometimes transferred to cloth and sewn into shirts that provide supernatural protection for those who do not want to be tattooed. Yan shirts are made in the seven lucky colors that correspond to the seven known planets. "Soldiers still use these magical shirts when going to battle," Sammy explains. "They wear yellow shirts on Mondays for long life, black shirts on Saturdays to make the enemy have fear!"

Magical Yantric astrological tattoo design.

The monk pauses on a page with the image of a leaping tiger. With a common ballpoint pen he starts to draw the tiger image onto Sammy's back between his shoulder blades. He chants quietly as he draws the design; Sammy sits meditatively with his eyes closed, hands to his chin. After a few minutes he is motioned over to an apprentice who has set up a small table with a crude tattoo machine, ink, and the clean needles. The ingredients of the tattoo ink are a closely guarded secret that supercharge the tattoo. Spirit oil, *Namman Prai,* has been taken from the chin of a recently dead person and added to the ink by the monk. Tattooers who specialize in aggressive and powerful tattoos mix a small amount of *Namman Prai* into the ink to increase the dangerous power of the tattoo. Sammy lies down on his stomach and the apprentice begins to tattoo. The young novice monks gather around, watching the tiger image take shape.

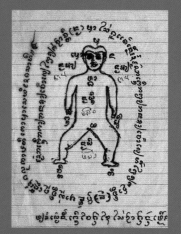

Longevity tattoo charm.

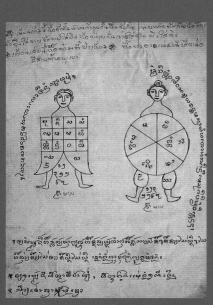

Tattoo charms from Monk's sketchbook.

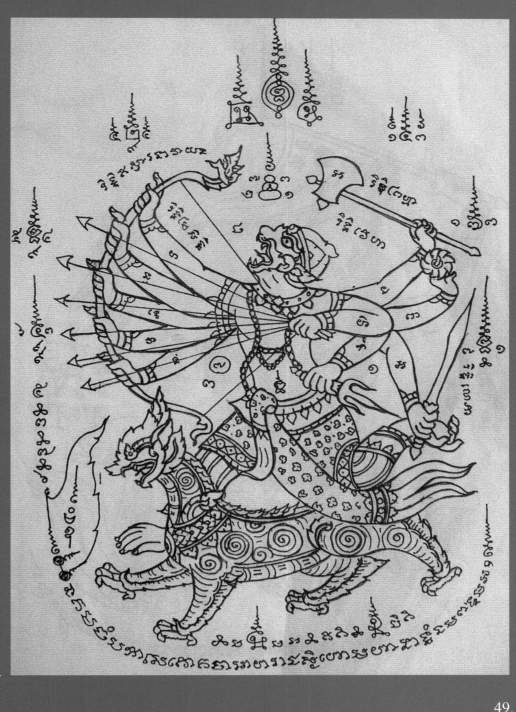

Tattoo charm of guardian deity riding lion.

49

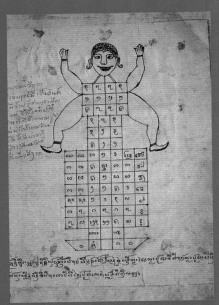

Yantric tattoo charm from Monk's sketchbook.

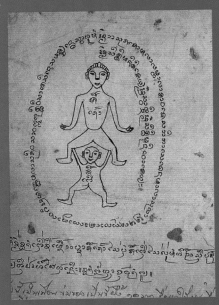

Tattoo charm for strength and health.

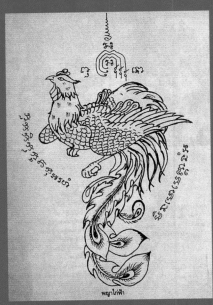

Peacock tattoo charm for good looks.

Tiger tattoo charms.

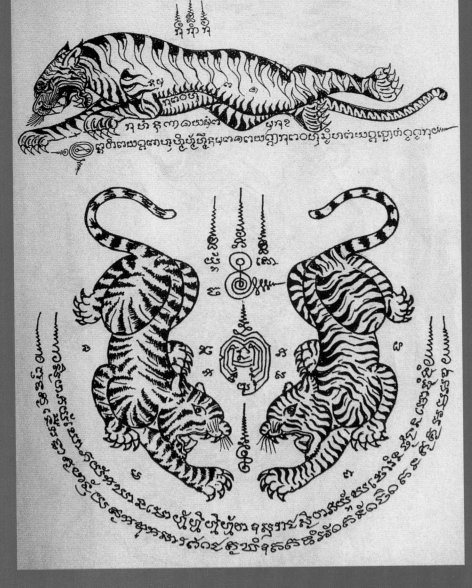

50

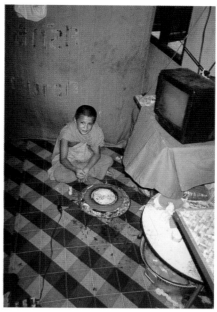

Novice monk sterilizing needles on hot plate.

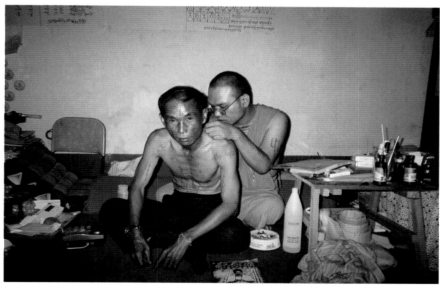

Monk drawing tiger design onto Sammy.

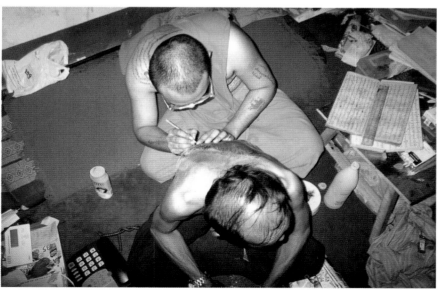

Monk drawing tiger design onto Sammy.

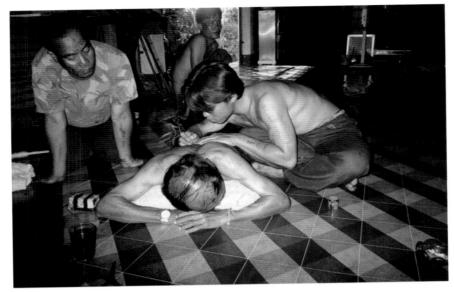

Apprentice tattooing tiger image.

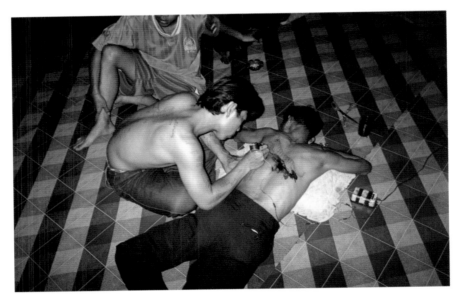

Apprentice tattooing tiger image.

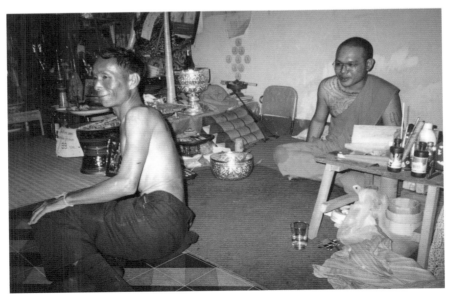

Monk blessing fresh tattoo.

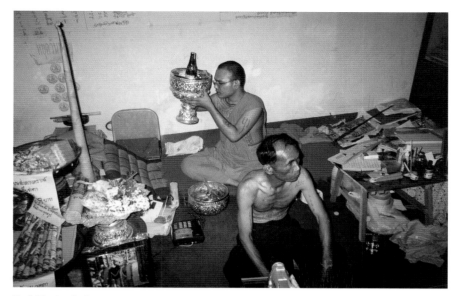

Monk blessing fresh tattoo.

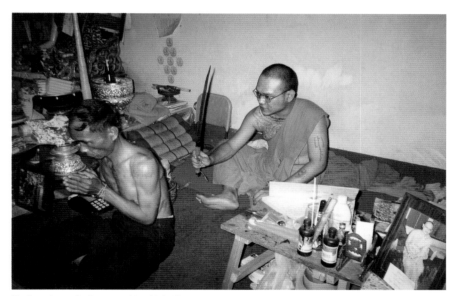

Monk cutting at fresh tattoo with spirit knife.

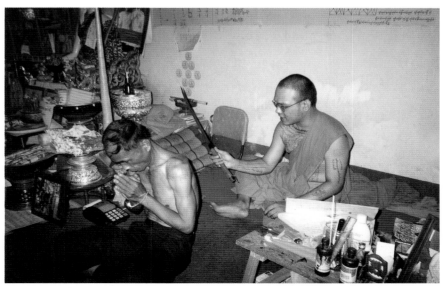

Monk cutting at fresh tattoo with spirit knife.

53

After an hour the apprentice has finished the tattoo and cleans Sammy's back of blood and ink. The monk motions him over to his side to complete the process, which will empower the tattoo by chanting a spell. Sammy sits facing forward and the monk wipes at the fresh tattoo, incanting a series of words. He then blows forcefully on the fresh tattoo that sends his psychic power into Sammy and awakens the tiger's animal spirit. The monk reaches into the shadows and pulls a long, antique spirit knife into view. The *Meed Phii* will be used by the monk to test the spells he has recited. As he continues to chant magical words, the monk raises the knife over the head of my unsuspecting driver and comes down hard onto the fresh tattoo. The sword hits with a loud thud and bounces back leaving a pronounced welt but no cut or blood. Sammy winces but continues to sit very still with his hands to his mouth as the monk comes down again with the long knife. There is another loud thud, a pronounced welt, but no cut or blood. The monk rears back but this time slashes to the side across my driver's right biceps that has no tattoo. The sword cuts deeply into the flesh and blood immediately flies from the large wound. Finally, the monk pulls back and stabs at Sammy's lower back near his kidneys, puncturing the skin. Sammy is completely rigid now and falls over like a tree onto his side. He is shaking violently but his hands are still together at his mouth.

It is hard to know why the monk has tested Sammy and the tattoo so forcefully and dramatically. The young novice monks haven't lifted an eye to any of it, the young apprentice who did the tattoo has been watching the kickboxing on the television and seems oblivious to the violent display. The monk looks at me almost defiantly, the expression in his eyes cold and emotionless. He has tested and illustrated his power and the authenticity of the tattoo.

Sammy rises slowly from his side. He looks dazed and possibly in a mild state of shock. Blood is running down his arm towards his hand and the welts on his back have taken a pronounced shape and turned bright red. He turns and bows in front of the monk, thanking him for the tattoo. The monk nods his head in recognition, points to the metal bowl and asks for an offering of some kind. Following protocol, Sammy gathers himself, willingly complies and puts some money in the bowl. His hands are shaking as he drops the offering into the bowl.

To maintain the tattoo's power, Sammy will have to follow rules. The monk talks to him, instructing about what is expected of his behavior. Sammy is told to limit his aggression and not to have too much sex. He should follow the five Buddhist precepts: No killing, stealing, lying, adultery, or drunkenness. The monk calls Sammy close and whispers into his ear. It is a secret mantra that Sammy will be able to recite to renew his tattoo's power.

Monk cutting at fresh tattoo with spirit knife.

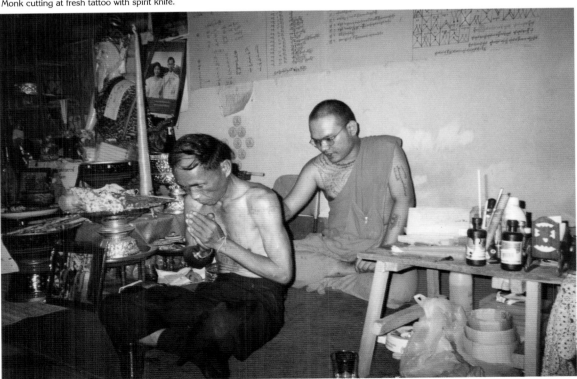

Chapter Four

In Search of the Tattooed Tiger Hunter

There had been a tiger attack two days before I arrived in Chiang Mai, Thailand. Very few of the big cats remain in the remote mountain region, but one had grabbed a hill tribe infant and dragged it into the thick cover of the jungle. The local newspaper said that the authorities were scouring the steep mountain trails, looking for what if anything was left of the child's remains. They were also looking for the cat; this was not the first time a small child had been snatched. A pattern was developing and suspicions were that the same cat was responsible for several deaths.

The attack came as a strange coincidence. I had traveled to the region from Bangkok to connect with a 4-wheel drive enthusiast club called the Chiang Mai Jungle Club. My friend George and his club were going to take me deep into the jungle towards the boarder of Myanmar (Burma) in search of an 86-year-old hill tribesman who had hunted tiger in his youth. He was tattooed with magical tiger charms that had brought him luck; finding him would make for a great adventure.

450 miles from Bangkok and 3000 feet above sea level, Chiang Mai is known as the Flower of the North. Life is slow and provincial compared to the Thai capital but the small city has experienced the steady encroachment of Western modernization during last 20 years. Signs for Pizza Hut, Mister Donuts, and McDonald's blend weirdly into the main street in the shadow of the 600-year-old Buddhist temple, Wat Phra Singh.

Wat Phra Singh

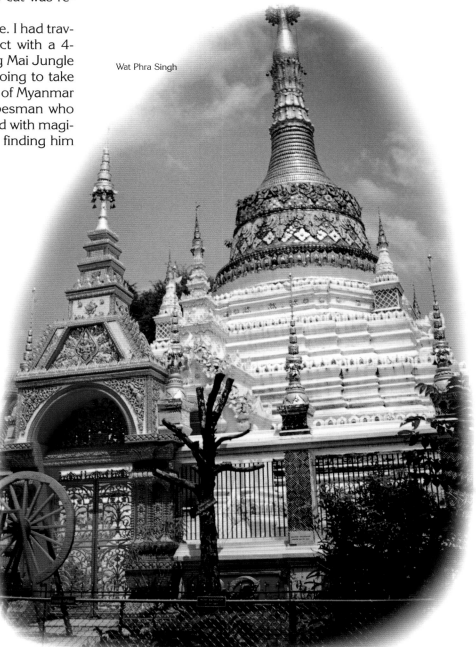

Peddle taxi man.

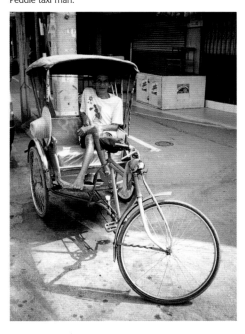

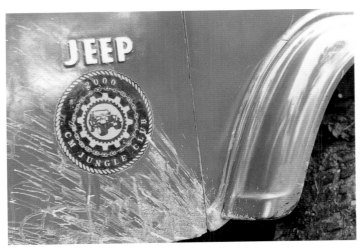
Chaing Mai Jungle Club jeep.

The mountainous territory from Chiang Mai to the Burmese and Laos boarder is called the Golden Triangle, or Sop Ruak in Thai. Powerful hill tribe warlords who cultivate the infamous poppy plant vigilantly control the region. Their private armies are funded with the proceeds from the opium they export on the world narcotics market. They are heavily armed with the latest in military hardware and nobody, including the Thai government, messes with them. The Shan, Lanna Thai, and Hmong Hill tribes populate the territory surrounding Chiang Mai. The long-necked Karen people live in the area to the northwest near the town of Mae Hong Son. Karen women are known for the copper rings they wear around their necks. Rings are added every 3 years during their early lives until they reach 21 years old and their necks become elongated by an inch or so. The tribe believes it is descendent from the God of the wind and the dragon, which the long necks are thought to imitate.

I rendezvous with George on a dusty Chiang Mai back street near a mechanic's garage. He is standing on the outcrop of his Jeep's front bumper, stooped over the huge engine, pulling at hoses. It is a short-wheel-based model from the late 1980s with a lot of clearance underneath. To protect the passengers from the baking sun, it has a canvas canopy roof stretched tight over the thick tubular roll bar. The other club members are gathered around their impressive vehicles, checking fluid levels, inspecting oversized leaf springs, and kicking at the monstrous tires. Everyone looks to be about the same age, somewhere in their early thirties. Each of the four Jeeps is pretty mean looking and they all have a paramilitary style about them: mud is caked on the sideboards, the winches on the front bumpers have heavy hooks and cables that have seen serious duty, the radio antenna are bent over and buttoned down. There are axes and shovels bolted to the back bumpers. Exterior air filters are mounted high, at windshield level.

Mechanic's garage.

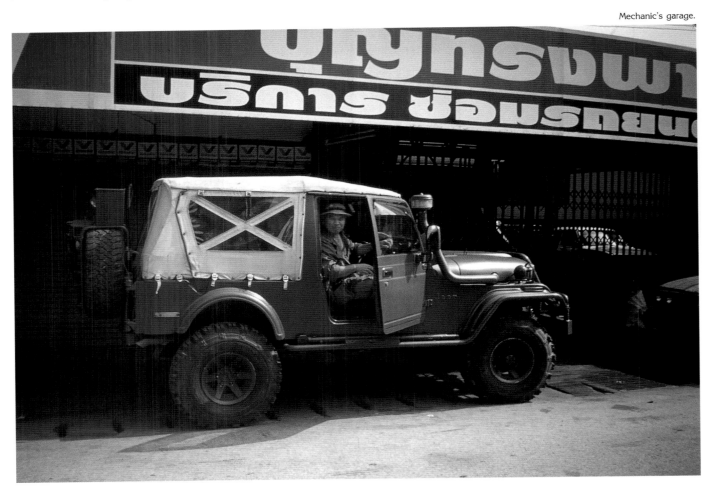

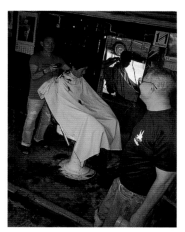

Sidewalk barber, Chiang Mai.

A half dozen Club members and two men who have been hired to scout the trails greet me warmly. A few speak English and tell me with excited smiles that they are looking forward to going "deep in-country" in search of the tattooed man. I look at the jacked-up, mud-covered jeeps and wonder how deep we are going... One of the guides takes the axes and starts working a sharpening file over them, the other guide is crisscrossing lengths of heavy chain around a Jeep's bumper. These people mean business... As the guide winds the chain, I notice he is heavily tattooed with protective amulets on his upper arms and chest.

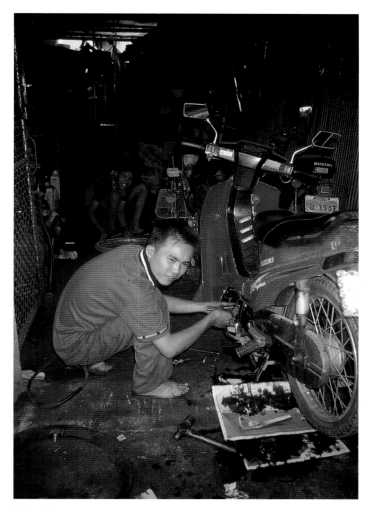

Mechanic's garage.

Guide with magical tattoos. Lord Brahma image in center of chest.

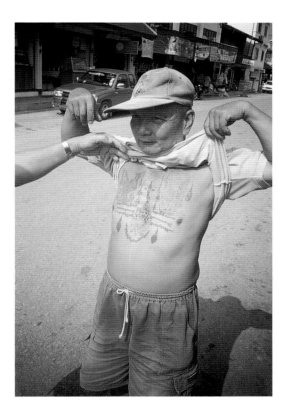

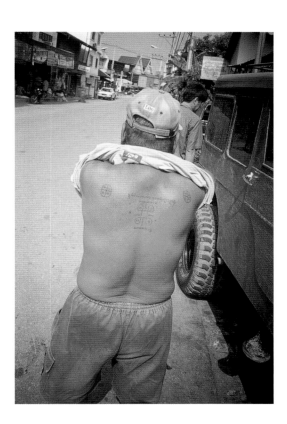

The small paved road out of Chiang Mai runs flat and then starts to climb and switch back into the mountains. The vegetation gets thicker as we climb, and the teak trees become larger. At the top of a rise George pulls over at a thatched roofed, roadside stand where women are selling different homegrown fruit. One approaches, pushing a plastic bowl full of squirming, puffy white grub worms at me. I decline but the guides pluck several from the bowl and pop them into their mouths with a chomp. They smile at me and swallow and I wonder again how far "in-country" we're going?

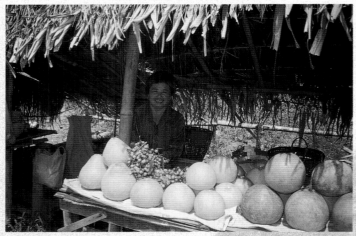

Roadside fruit stand.

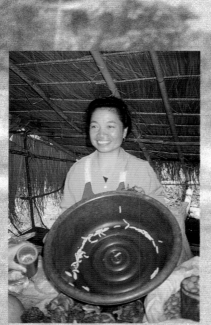

Woman with fresh grubs.

Road out of Chaing Mai.

A few miles from the stand George takes an abrupt left down a set of tire tracks that run into the thick green cover. Everyone stops for a moment and secondary gearboxes grind and settle. George dumps his clutch whipping our necks and his engine changes mood from a purr to a menacing growl. Each time he hits the gas, the Jeep punches ahead, chewing through the apron growth of the jungle as we begin to climb. In a few minutes we are surrounded by very heavy jungle vegetation — big palms splay out under the teak tree canopy that is 40 feet above our heads. George tells me over the roar of his engine that this used to be tiger country 30 years ago, but development has chased the last cats inland. The intense vegetation limits my view to 20 feet and I wonder how it has changed over the years. The teak seem tall and densely grouped, there is nobody or anything vaguely development-like in sight; just green leafy stuff everywhere growing out of orange colored soil. The tiger newspaper story scrolls through my memory.

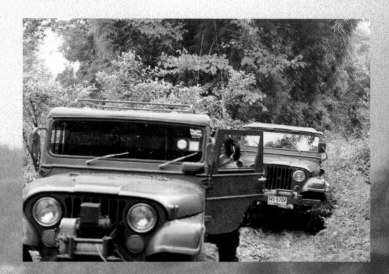

Vehicles moving into the jungle.

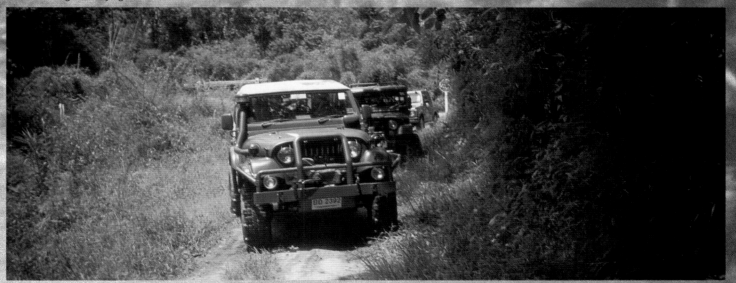

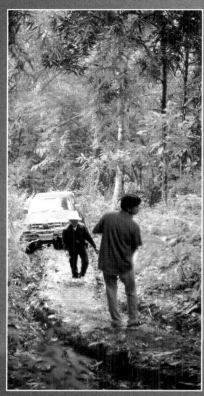

Walking back down the trail.

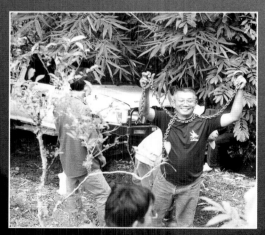

Preparing the chains.

George downshifts as the grade steepens and the Jeep gets aggressive. We are beginning to pitch upwards and it becomes necessary to hold on to the roll bar that arcs overhead. The trail has narrowed to an overgrown footpath, small tree branches smack at the windshield and swipe at us from the side. I look behind at the other Jeeps and notice just how steep our trail has become. They are tossing around beneath us, grabbing at the clay soil, trying to stay on the path. As we climb, the mountain ridge emerges from behind us. The intense green of the vegetation is diffused through thick mist that hangs in the trees. Everything looks

The view from up on the ridge.

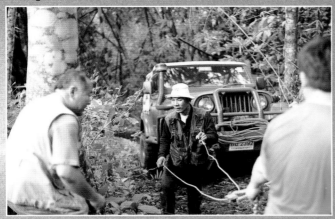

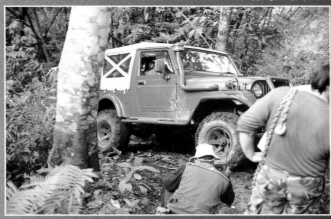

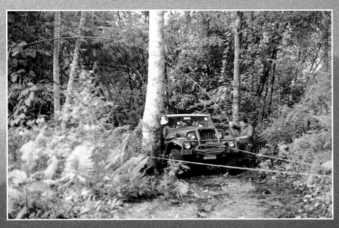

Winding winch cable around the teak trees.

We have been at it for more than an hour and are now way up on the ridge. The heat and humidity is increasing as we get deeper into the jungle and George warns of insects dropping from the foliage. Many are parasites that will attach themselves and suck your blood. He describes a little black inchworm that looks harmless, but will lay its eggs in you. As it bites an anesthetic is injected, so you never knew what hit you until the thousands of eggs hatch under your skin... Our tires start to slip and we are thrown to the edge of the trail. George spins the wheel, dodging foot deep washout ruts created by rain runoff. The path zigzags up the ridge and George points towards a level area where we will eat lunch. From below, a Jeep horn blasts and George hits the brakes — somebody is stuck.

We unlash the shovels and stumble back down the steep trail. The guides are chopping at small trees and letting out the cable from the winch at the front of the stranded Jeep. It has fallen into a series of 3-foot deep ruts and is sunk up to the axles. Everyone knows the drill: people are throwing the chopped wood into the ruts to even out the grade. One guide has walked the cable to a big teak tree and looped it around. The other guide has attached a length of chain to the Jeep and hooked it onto another winch cable at a different angle. This job is going to take the power of two winches to get things moving. I follow George's lead and start to dig at the ruts, caving them onto the chopped wood. It is really hot; sweat immediately saturates my T-shirt and I feel like I am working inside a blazing pizza oven. Everyone stands back as the guides push at their winch's hand-held remote switches. The powerful motors make a whirring sound and as everything tight- ens, the cabled tree groans and pops. The Jeep driver stamps the gas peddle to the floor, spraying mud into the sky and the vehicle pops free like a child's toy. He navigates it over the chopped wood towards the more stable trail shoulder and kills the engine. There are two more Jeeps to steer past the trouble spot and then a break for lunch.

Towards the end of lunch one of the guides pushes a small container of black pasty stuff at me. I ask what it is and George translates that they will tell me after I eat it… I take a pinch of sticky rice, daub a chunk of the black paste, and pop it in. Oh shit… My eyes immediately start tearing and my tongue ignites. As I swallow, the guide volunteers over his laughter that I have just eaten crushed, fermented land crab that is prepared, buried, and aged with green and red chili peppers for several months… I like spicy food and take another serving to the wide-eyed surprise of everyone. Surviving the challenge, I wipe the last of the sticky rice from my mouth as everyone breaks down lunch camp. George has keyed his Jeep and is waiting for me to climb on board. It is early afternoon and we have a way to go until we reach the old man's village.

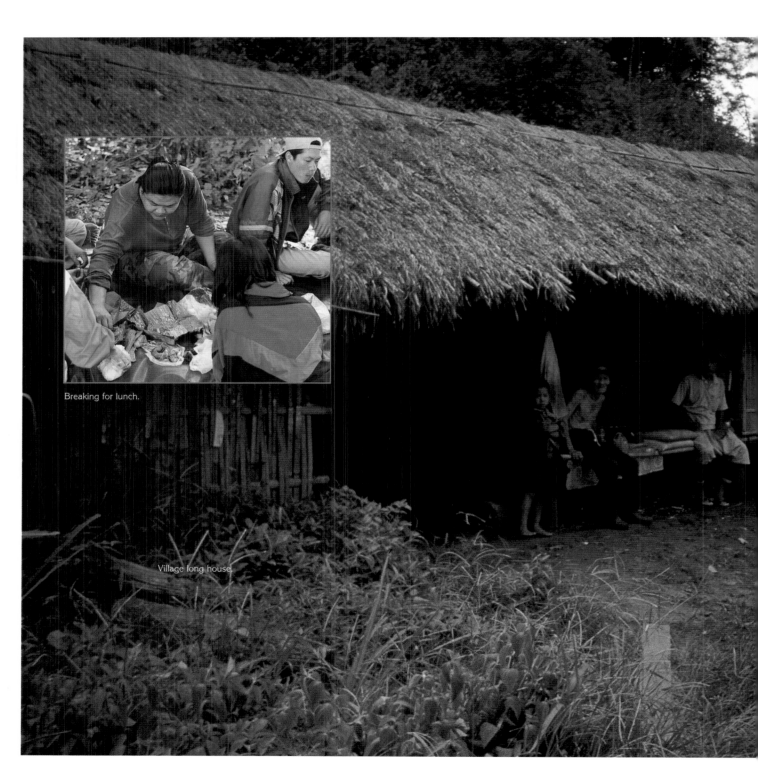

Breaking for lunch.

Village long house.

62

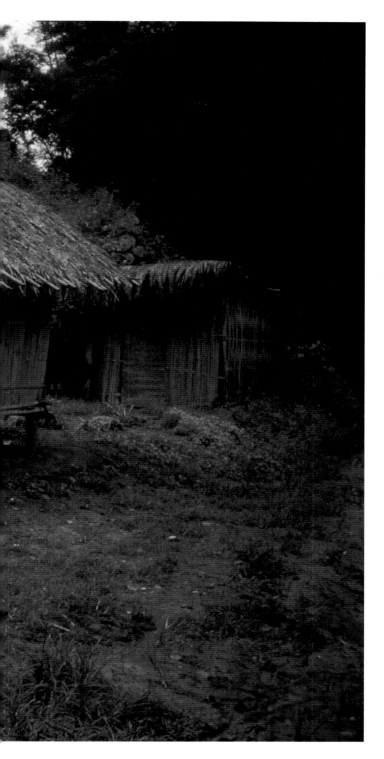

After another 45 minutes of bouncing our way across the ridge, the trail widens and seems more traveled. We emerge from the thick foliage into a very small village that is nested next to a mild stream. There are two or three thatched roofed long houses, 12 feet long and 8 to 10 feet wide, propped up on short stilts. A few dogs quickly greet our caravan, tails frozen in guarded apprehension. They are quiet but their curled lips and intense eyes say they are ready for anything. George advises me not to touch the dogs when we get out… There are three middle-aged women standing knee-deep in the stream doing laundry. They lift their heads to measure us as we approach and finally offer cautionary smiles. Three young boys walk timidly through the stream towards us wearing soccer jerseys. Their eyes are warm but aware. A young man walks onto the narrow porch of one of the long houses and waves in greeting. The look on everyone's face says that they see very few outsiders here.

Entering the village.

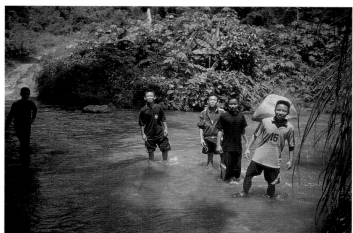

Entering the village.

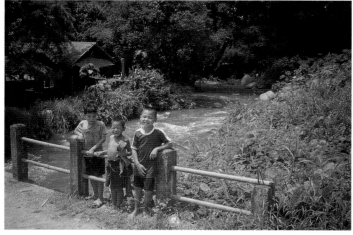

63

One of our guides talks to the hill tribe people in their Thai dialect, asking if the tiger hunter is here. The man on the porch nods and gestures inside his house, waving us over. He calls inside and a very thin old man wearing a brown felt hat emerges, takes a seat on the porch and looks at us. He is tattooed on his arms, back, chest, and shoulders with small faded amulets of pouncing tigers that dance around his body in a subtle pattern. His skin is dark from the sun, wrinkles bunch up at his elbows and knees. From under the brim of his hat, he looks at us with mild curiosity, a bit shocked to see inquisitive outsiders staring at him. The three boys from the stream move over to him, sitting near like he is their grandfather. They slowly glide their gentle eyes past the old man towards us, wondering. The women have resumed beating their clothes into the water.

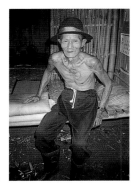

Tiger hunter.
Note small tiger image tattoos.

Through our guide, George asks the man how old he is and about hunting tiger. He waves his hand, responding that he is 86 years old and that there are very few tiger left. They are old like him and live deep in the jungle, hiding. George asks when he hunted and the old man replies he hunted when he was young. Tigers would attack their villages, taking the children and the dogs and he would have to retaliate. That was his job, to challenge the tigers and protect the village.

George continues, asking about his tattoos and the man explains that hunting tiger was very dangerous. The cats knew you were looking for them. They would wait for you in the bush, let you to pass and then come up behind you and kill you. You had no chance with them; they were the best hunters. You were dead before you could scream. He moves his hands in a violent ripping motion, pulsing his fingers like big claws, gesturing that they would tear you to shreds. He continues, saying that the tattoos were the only thing that protected him from the cats. As he speaks, the young boys become quiet and their smiles drop away to nothing. They look for our reaction to the old man's explanation as I twist around calmly, peering into the surrounding thick jungle. Without the roar of the jeeps it is very quiet, just the movement of the stream slipping past.

Through George I ask the old man who tattooed him and he replies that village priests had tattooed him. It was all passed down over the years; the designs were generations old. He continues, pointing at the young boys that they will not receive tiger tattoos; there are no more tigers to hunt. The boys look at him with resignation, hunching their shoulders shyly. I ask how this makes him feel, experiencing the end of the tiger. He sits calmly, looking at me, then at the others in our group and finally at the oversized Jeeps that have turned his front yard into a parking lot... His eyes stay fixed on the Jeeps and he says nothing. There is an awkward silence for a few minutes and then he rises slowly and walks back into his long house. It is hard to know if he is tired, bored, or upset.

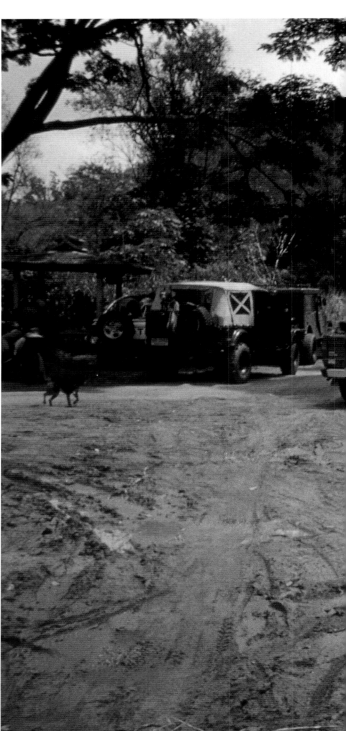

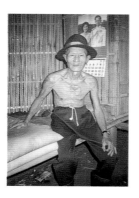
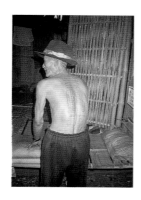

The intensity of the sun is fading as the afternoon matures and George suggests we get back on the trail. It will be dark before we make it back to Chiang Mai and traveling in the jungle after sundown is dangerous. Too much can go wrong, even if there aren't many tigers left... We all clasp our hands in front of our chins and say thank you to the people remaining on the porch. As we pass the stream on out way out of the village, the women are corkscrewing their laundry, wringing out the water. They raise their heads as we pass, smile mildly and return to their work.

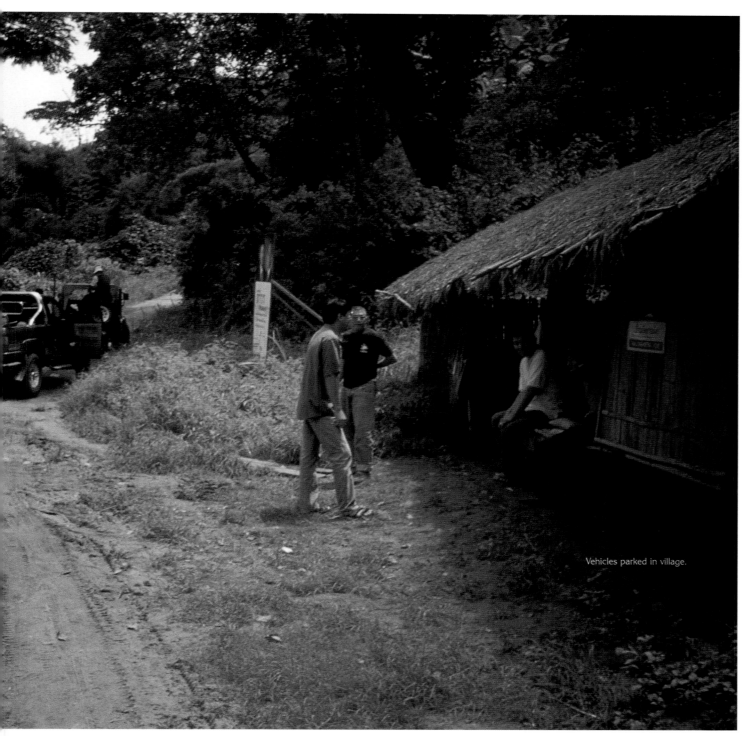

Vehicles parked in village.

65

Chapter Five

Wat Bang Phraw
The Temple of Thai Buddhist Tattoo

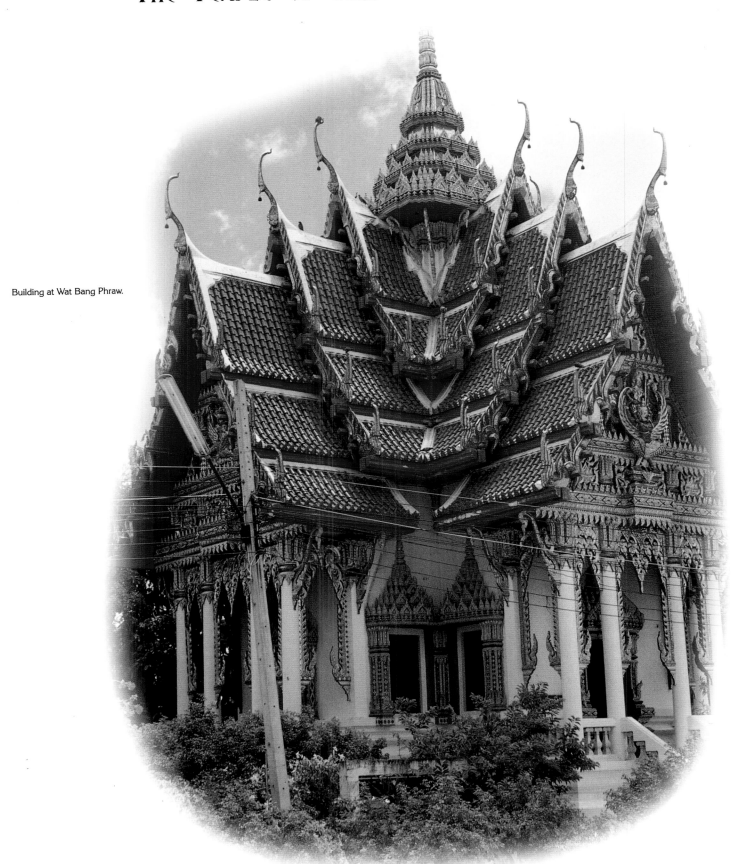

Building at Wat Bang Phraw.

The hectic and dangerous Bangkok traffic fades as we drive northwest from the city limits. The land runs flat and the edges of the small scale, two-lane highway are flanked with strip mall type businesses: auto repair shops, restaurants, and an occasional glitzy massage parlor. Ten miles out all this also fades into big leafy palms and scrub tropical growth. Ramshackle, nondescript, cinder block buildings spring up every 100 yards along the road edge. Slower traffic of small motorcycles pulls to the left as we pass. Each bike has two or three passengers and the women are riding sidesaddle. Smoky fires burn in clearings at the jungle's edge, pushing back its voracious spread. Red clay soil contrasts the bold green hue of the vegetation.

My guide Kevin and I are headed about 50 clicks (km) out of Bangkok towards the Nakhon Chai Sri region where the tattoo temple compound, Wat Bang Phraw, is located. *Wat* is Thai for temple and always precedes a temple's formal name. We have both resigned ourselves to getting lost a bunch, the signs are few and the temple is not listed on any map. The only people who know about it are the Thai people who gather there to receive traditional, curative and magical tattoos from the monks. Kevin speaks Thai and we are hoping that we'll find our way. A few days earlier, Jimmy Wong, who tattoos in Bangkok, had drawn a map for us to follow and he wrote down a few distinct mile markers to keep our eyes peeled for. As the occasional road sign flies by, I look at the illegible curlicue Thai script and wonder if we are blowing past an important turn.

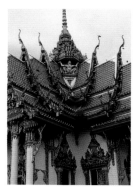

Building at Wat Bang Phraw.

After an hour we reach a small town with a perplexing "Y" intersection. I wonder, which way — right or left? Kevin pulls over next to a group of men who are sitting in the shade, under a building outcrop. They turn to look at us — just curious, all smiles, nothing threatening. Thailand is a deeply Buddhist country; aggression, anger, and threat does not have a place in the mindset of the people. "Koh-to-na-kop, sawat-dee-kop." Excuse me, hello, Kevin says to the men. "Wat Bang Phraw?" As the men gather around the car window I show the tattoos on my left arm. Smiles sprout across their faces as they try to decipher my ink. People in Thailand like tattoos. It is a part of their life in a very natural way. In unison, they all nod their heads and point to the left down the road. One man shakes his hand encouragingly, as if to say not too far away, keep going. I thank the men, "Kop-Khun-Mana-Kop" and make a mental note of what this place looks like. We are going to have to find our way home too.

The temple complex is impressive. Exotic white buildings with steeply peaked roofs are arranged near each other. The rooflines of a few of the buildings are painted with gold leaf that shimmers in the hot sun. There are statuettes of Buddhist deities in the crotches of the roof angles. The trim around the windows is painted in a deep maroon red, gold, and dark blue — everything looks otherworldly. We notice that in the rear of the complex there is an old stucco building with a front porch and steps. Twenty or so stray dogs are sitting on the steps or wandering around sniffing at each other. They are underfed and mangy looking but seem friendly enough, wagging their corkscrew tails in short cautionary jabs.

Front door at Wat Bang Phraw.

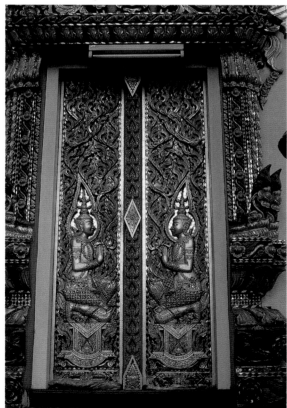

Front steps of tattoo building.

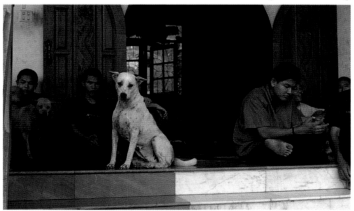

A few dozen younger and middle-aged men are sitting on the porch and steps in the shade; talking quietly, waiting turn to be tattooed. Several have necklaces of dangling charms that are contained in small plastic coverings. It is hot out — South East Asian sticky-hot that makes your clothes feel like clinging, damp dish rags. We remove our shoes and walk up the short rise of stairs onto the veranda. One monk is out on the porch surrounded by four or five youths that are stretching the skin of a friend's back. Another monk is inside a dark room with ancient, stained walls. There is an altar in the room with flowers arranged around a central Buddha. Incense and candles are burning. As we enter, I notice the long needle stick the monk is working into a young man's back makes a squishing sound as it hits the skin. The room has a heavy, almost oppressive smell of body odor, mildew, and stray dog. Everyone looks up at us as we enter. I cup my palms to my face, bow slightly, and say, "Sawat-dee-kop." The young men cup their palms and return the hello. They are curious; a few seem mildly suspicious — very few if any Westerners visit here. Everyone is very polite. Thai people are very gentle and very polite.

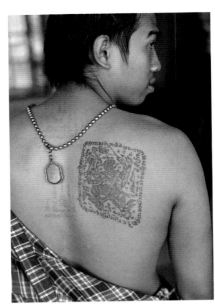

Tattoo devotee at Wat Bang Phraw.

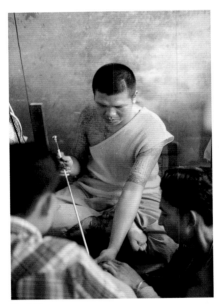

Monk Ya.

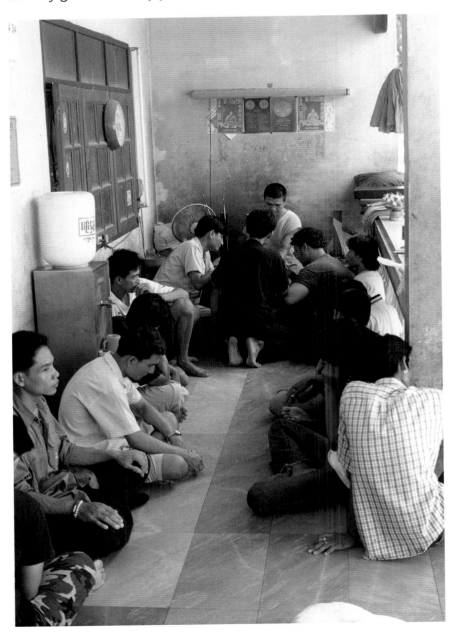

Tattoo devotees with monk Ya.

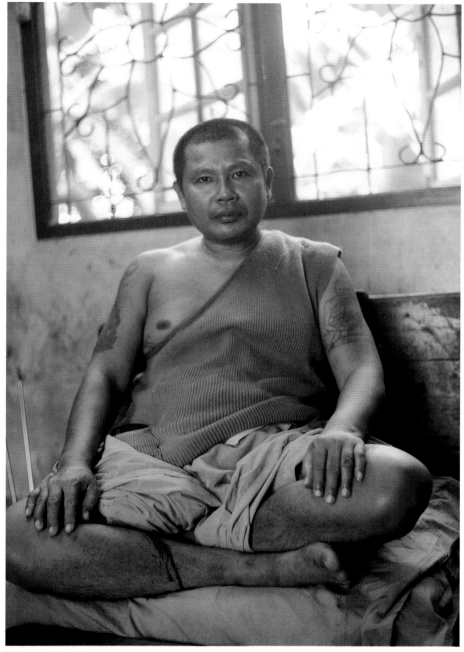

Senior monk Sam-Pun.

Monk Ya working.

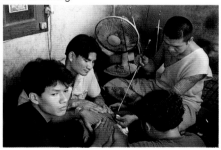

Monk Ya working.

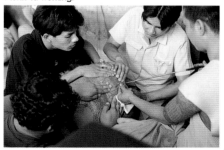

Monk Sam-Pun tattooing.

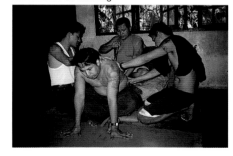

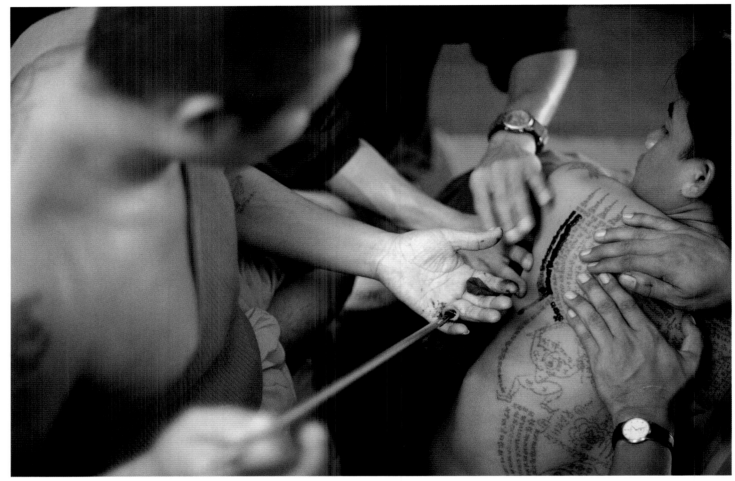
Stretching skin for monk Sam-Pun.

In the rear of the room a middle-aged monk sits cross-legged near the large central alter display, dressed in a bright saffron orange robe. He is working on the center of a young man's back, gently pushing at a charcoal transfer of a charm design with his long needle stick. The long metal wand-like stick has a sharpened, tooled tip that has slits in it. The oil or ink runs down the tip almost like a fountain pen. The monk is not tattooing with ink; after 20 or so hits he dips the needles into a small ceramic cup that has an inch of orange tinted vegetable oil in it. The oil has been anointed and blessed by the monks. Without ink, the needles will leave a slight scar of the symbol, not a distinct black image. As the monk pushes at the design with his needles, he is pushing power and protection into the young man's body and psyche. There is a deep sense of calm in the room among the others who are waiting to be tattooed. No one is talking; they just sit cross-legged, watching and waiting. A few stray dogs wander around sniffing at the corners of the room before slinking out onto the porch where a dozen young men sit in the shade waiting turn.

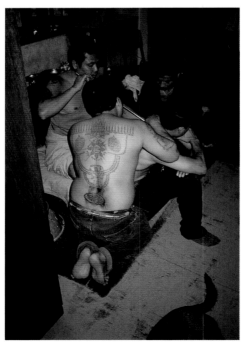
Stretching skin.

70

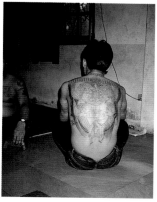

Tattoo by monk Sam-Pun.

At the end of the stone porch a younger monk decorated with running script on his shoulders and arms sits encircled by six youths who are preparing a design block to make a transfer. One youth is lighting and adjusting a small Bunsen-like burner that consists of a bottle full of alcohol with a thick cotton wick. Another is preparing a carved wooden tablet, carefully wiping camphor oil over the relieved surface. He positions the surface over the mild flame, moving the wood back and forth, peeking occasionally to make sure carbon is being produced over all the design.

Carbonizing wooden block for transfer.

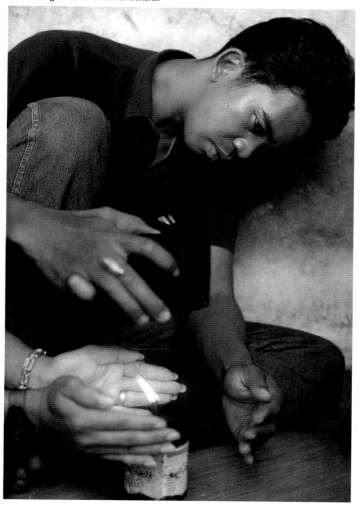

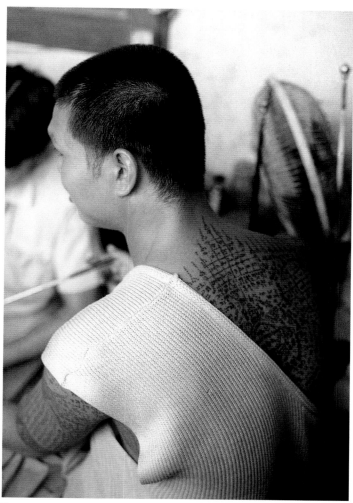

Monk Ya

71

Nearby on a stone banister there are a dozen or so carved wooden design tablets. The blocks are old, possibly very old. The patina of the wood is dark, shiny and rich from years of oil and flame. There are images of the Monkey King, curling snakes, magical monograms, and outstretched leaping tigers. The tiger seems to be the most popular. Most of the seated men have one tattooed on their chest. The senior monk who is the patron of this temple and now close to 90 years old, has a wide reputation he established early for his ability to quell the power of the tiger. Legend has it that he has the ability to calm, mount, and ride wild tigers — quieting them with his meditative energy.

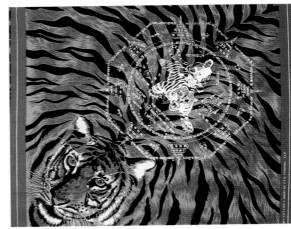

Fabric charm with monk Bun.

Painting with head monk Bun.

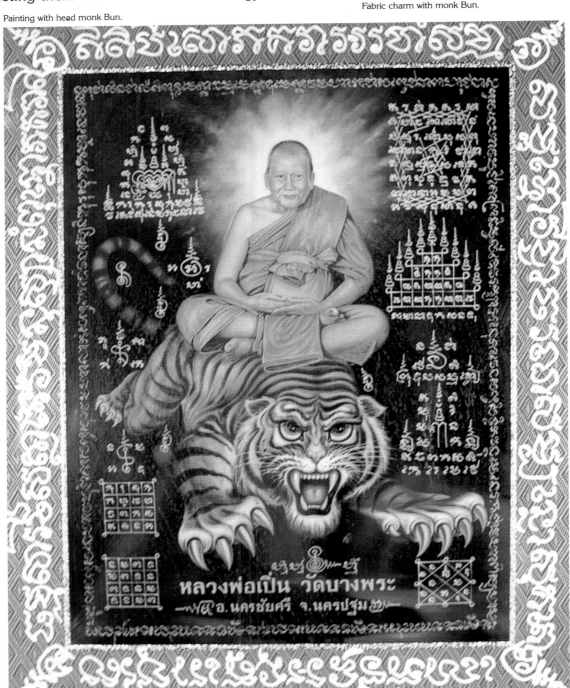

72

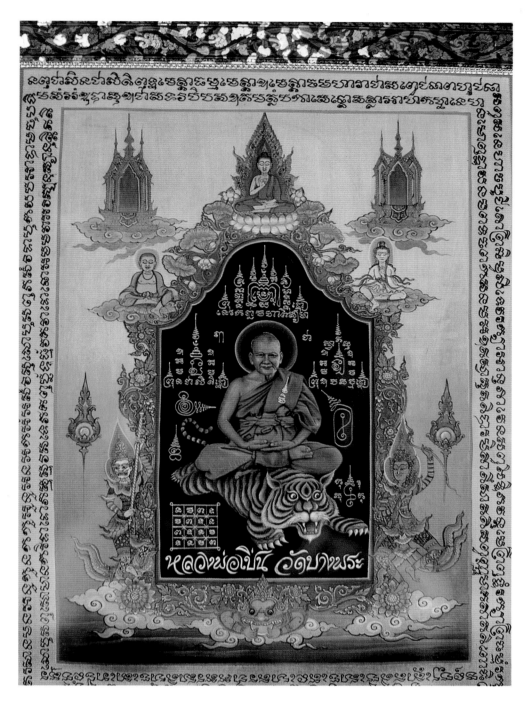

Painting with head monk Bun.

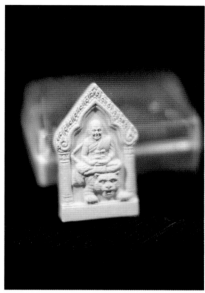

Magical clay amulet of monk Bun riding tiger.

Wooden blocks for transfer; Hanuman (L) Khmer Lion (R).

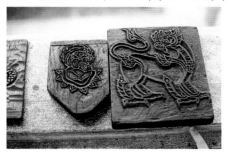

Leaping tiger transfer block.

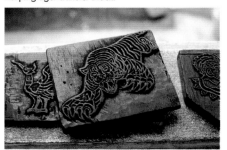

Wooden transfer blocks; Hanuman (R).

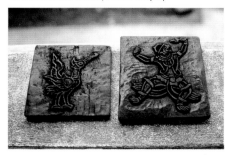

We ask a few of the seated men about their tiger charm tattoo, pointing at the small Thai script that is surrounding the contour of the image. They tell us that they wear the image for power, that it is helpful to them in their life. The tiger image represents the spirit of the senior monk and his ability to calm the dangerous power of the animal. The image is obviously a metaphor for the path these men have chosen to take during their life. It is interwoven with deep Buddhist faith in the ability of meditative, calm energy to produce positive results.

The other tattoos the men wear are cryptic — running script on their arms and small talismans on the shoulder blades. I have heard that some of the symbols are very direct in their meaning, preventing drowning and illness, neutralizing enemies, conjuring a love interest.

Some of the talismans make the wearer bulletproof or uncuttable with sharp blades. I point to one man's tattoo, make a cutting gesture and shake my hand as if so say, *can't cut*. He smiles and points to another of his tattoos, pulls his finger across it like a knife blade and then shakes his finger to say *can't cut*. The tattoo image is magical: it has pretty curlicue caps at the top and some script arranged in a boxlike shape. Some of these charms date back to the ancient Indochinese Khmer culture established around the year 500 A.D. The exact meanings have been lost through the ages, but devout faith in their power persists. I notice that there are few if any tattoos below the waist. Images of Buddha and the Bodisattvas are not to be worn below the waist.

Heavily tattooed temple devotee.

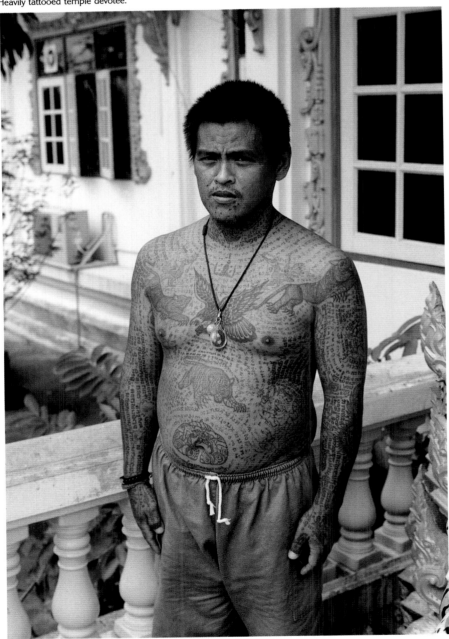

Monk Ya.

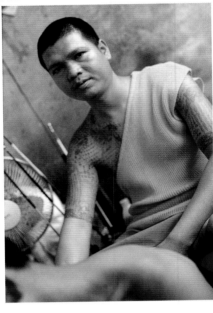

Magical tattoo with Jing-Joks, tiger and Hanuman.

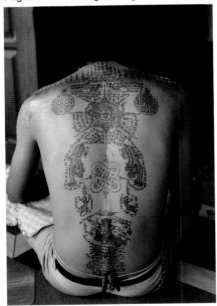

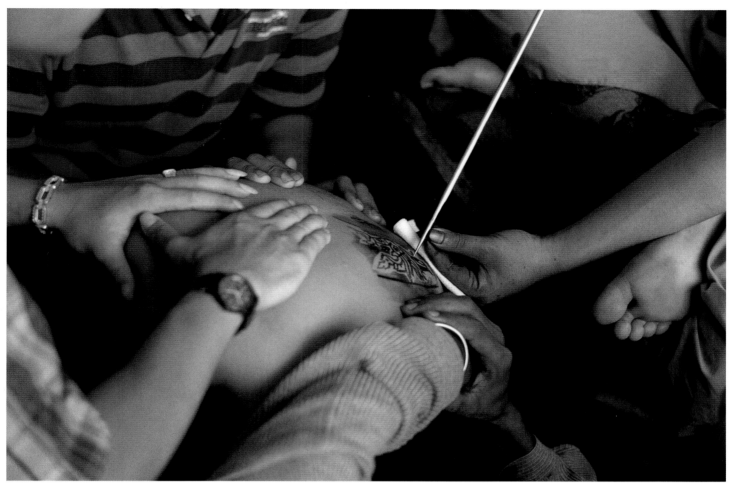

Monk Ya tattooing.

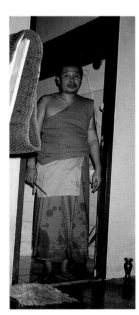

Monk Sam-Pun.

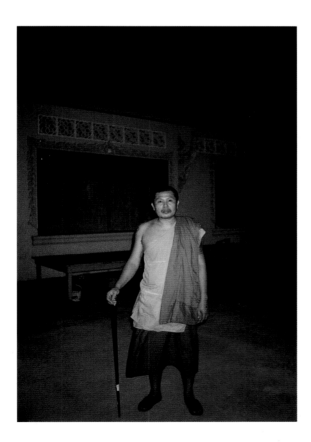

It is hard to break through into a deeper appreciation of what is happening here. I definitely feel like an intruder, although I am not being treated like one. The Thais have been practicing magical and protective tattooing for centuries. Wat Bang Phraw has been a part of this tradition for a long time. Standing on the temple veranda, watching monks tattoo the young men is so exotic to my western eyes. Tattooing in the West has been reduced to a trendy fad. There is still magic and power inherent in the process — people get tattooed in the West because they are looking for answers to big, unanswerable questions. The tattoo provides a possible link to the answer if you let it, but so much has been trivialized and marginalized, taken over by shallow, pop-cultural impulses. Watching the monks and young men sitting in the temple is a unique glimpse into the core power that makes people need to be tattooed.

75

The average age of the young men who are waiting their turn is somewhere in the early twenties. This is similar to what you might see in a tattoo shop in the West: a room full of young men waiting to get their first or second tattoo. A rite of passage in any culture, defining a moment in time. The big difference here is the magical nature of the designs and the status of the person doing the work. In any religion from Buddhism to Catholicism, priests are schooled, ordained intermediaries between two worlds: the sacred world of deep religious faith and the secular day-to-day world. In a very real way for the believers, priests have special powers to act as mediators and channels between a higher, intangible and complex religious entity like a God or Buddha and the common person. The young men who are being tattooed by the monks are willfully receiving a transferal of power from the monk. The tattoo image, the oil or ink, the pain and permanence, is the physical representation of that power and faith. This is a serious ritual intended to improve, affirm, and underscore the life of the young man who wears the tattoo. The purpose can be as secular as wanting to become bulletproof or uncuttable, or extremely esoteric and intangible. It is all magic.

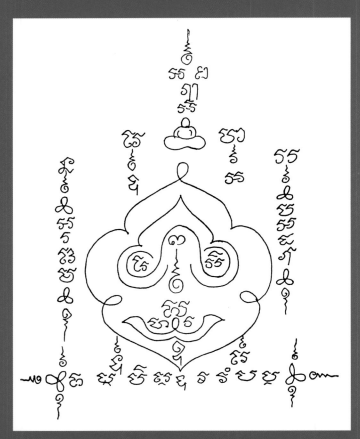

Magical tattoo design for eternal health

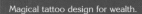

Magical tattoo design for wealth.

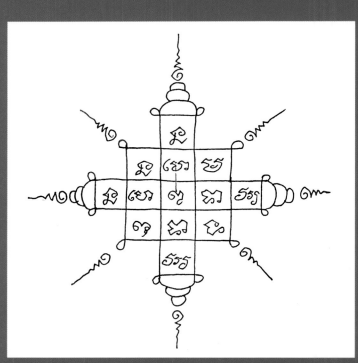

Magical tattoo design for prosperity.

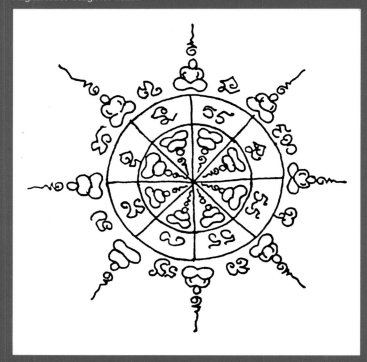

76

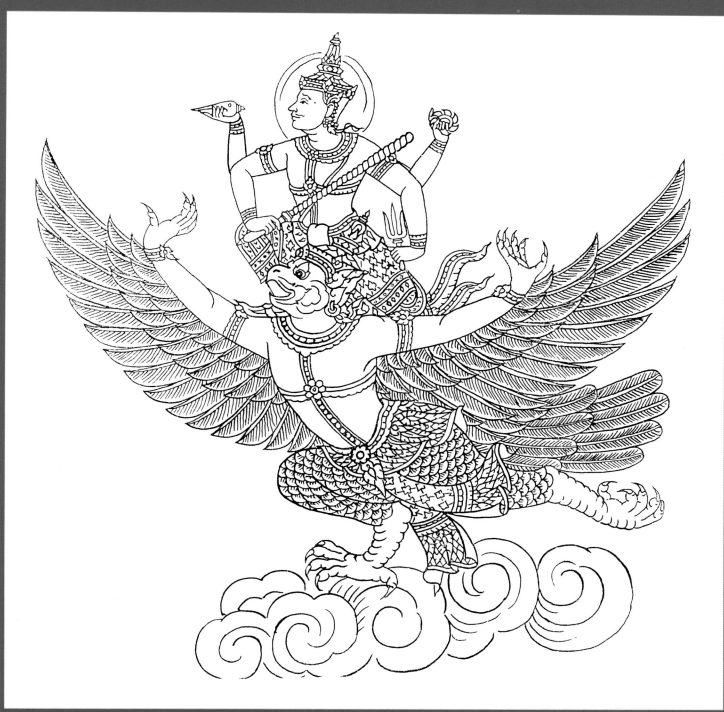

Tattoo design of Garuda and Vishnu.

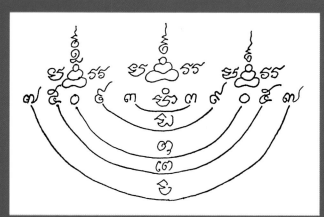

Magical tattoo design for power.

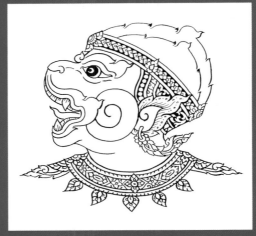

Tattoo design of Hanuman the Monkey King.

Tattoo design of Hanuman the Monkey King.

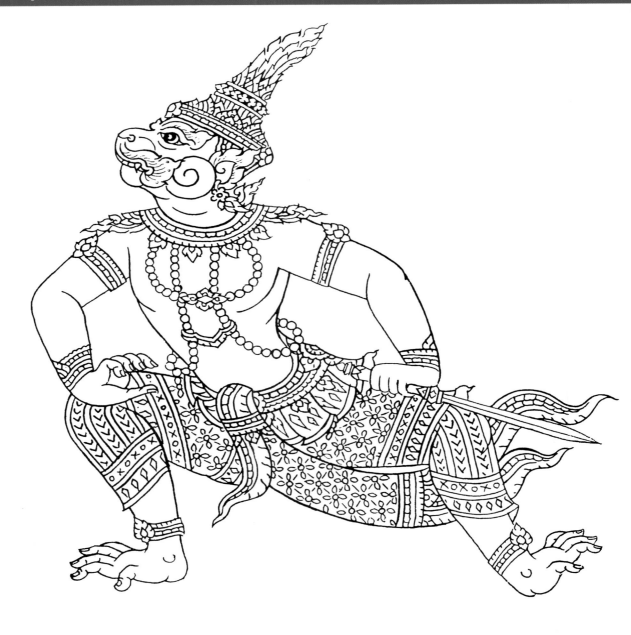

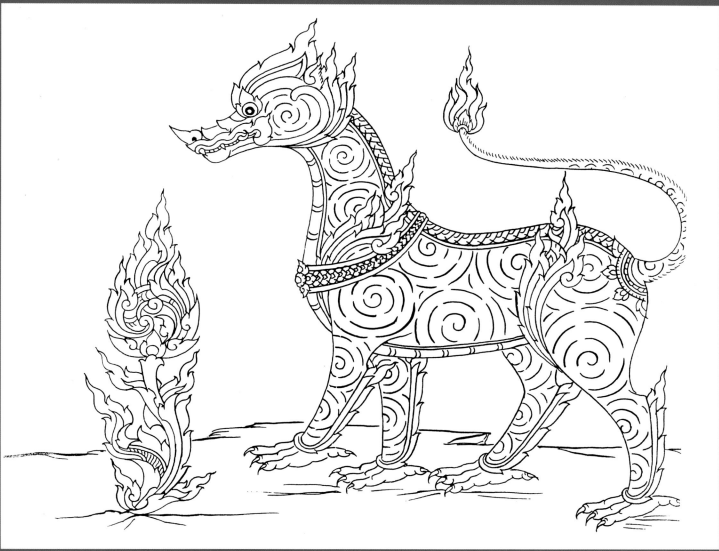

Tattoo design of Khmer Lion.

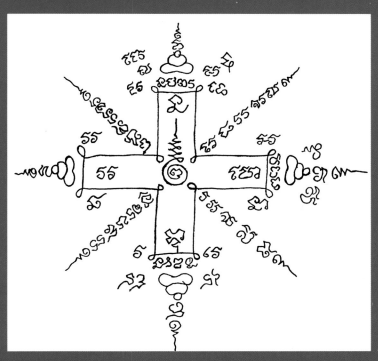

Magical tattoo design for attracting success.

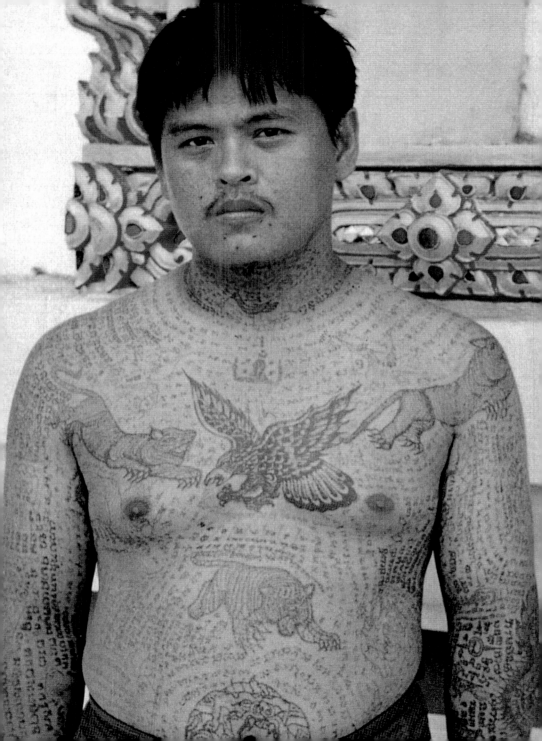

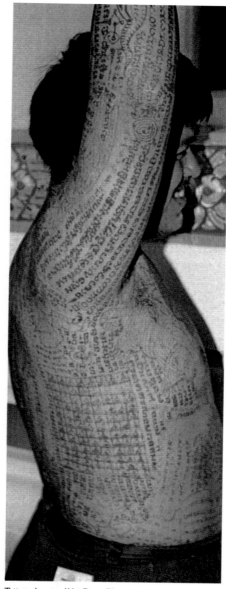

Tattoo devotee Wat Bang Phraw.

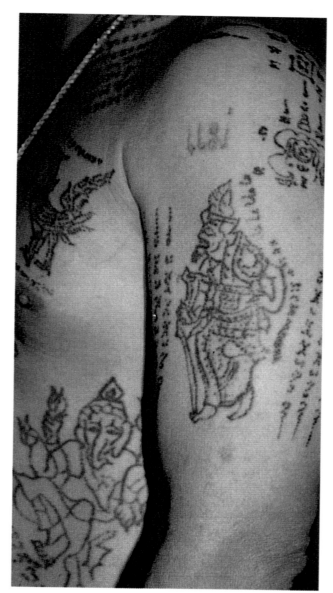

Tattoos Wat Bang Phraw. Note Ruesi on arm and Ganesha on ribs.

There are no women to be seen and I wonder if women get tattooed at all or to the extent that men do. Thai Buddhist monks are not supposed to touch women in any way and I wonder if this prohibition prevents the accessibility to the practice for Thai women.

We are led by a temple official from the tattoo area towards an administrative-like building that has two cast statues of tigers at the door. The senior monk is sleeping, but his direct subordinate would like to see us. Shoes off again, we are taken up a few flights of stairs to a larger room that has a golden Buddha and alter at the front. There is a rich, red carpet covering the floor at the altar. When you enter a room like this, it is customary to kneel at the alter, sitting back on your heels, cup your hands and bow forward, holding your hands so your fingertips are at your forehead. It is good to repeat this bowing process a few times in respect.

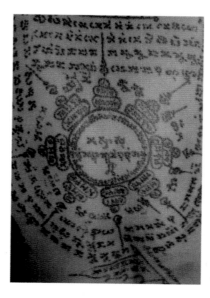

Tattoos, Wat Bang Phraw.

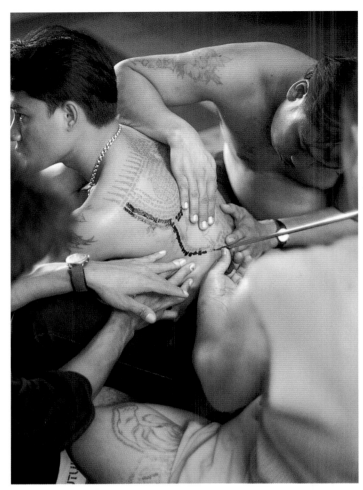

Tattooing, Wat Bang Phraw.

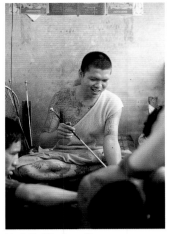

Monk, Wat Bang Phraw.

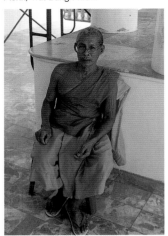

Monk Ya, Wat Bang Phraw.

The monk appears and ushers us into his office. We kneel a few feet away; careful to keep our feet properly positioned, pointing away from him. He projects a calm, respectful mood and asks why we have come. My friend interprets as I answer that I am a tattooer and a writer in New York City who has come to see the tattooing at the temple. The monk smiles and thanks me for my interest. He directs a subordinate to give me several bound booklets that will help me in my project. They are all written in curlicue Thai script. The monk asks to see my tattoos and squints at the work on my arms, nodding in appreciation of the Buddhist script I have. He blesses us, whispering a long series of sentences in a voice that oscillates high and low. I raise my hands to my forehead and say, Kop-Khun-Mana-Kop — thank you very much.

The sun is setting as we walk through the temple grounds, heading towards the car. The sky has gone dusk-purple, the moon is out and the heat of the day is fading. From one of the temple buildings the distinct, solitary sound of a monk chanting a series of incantations echoes through the old structures. He recites the long evening prayers in an unwavering, calm, monotone. A few dogs see us off, sniffing around the car as we pull away.

Tattoo devotee Wat Bang Phraw.

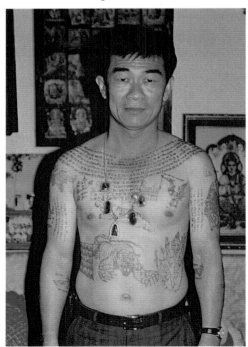

Tattoos, Wat Bang Phraw.

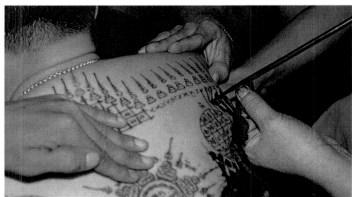

Chapter Six
CAMBODIA

KHMER MYTHOLOGY AND THE FOUNDATIONS OF INDOCHINA TATTOO

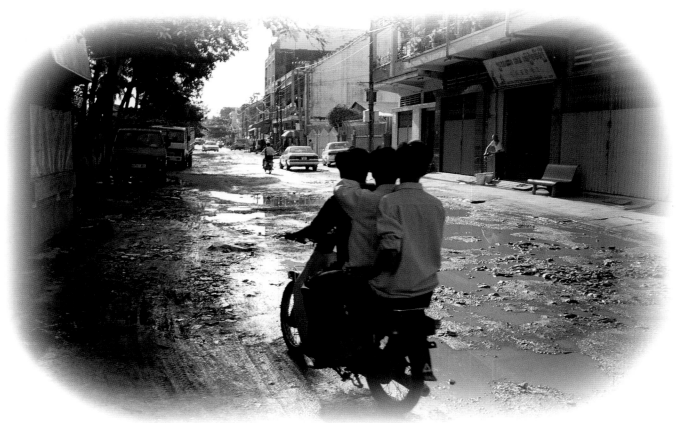

Phnom Penh street.

The gentle flow of motorbikes that dance around the battered, potholed streets of the Cambodian capital of Phnom Penh, begins to dry up with the setting sun. Young women with their hair pulled back out of the wind, sit three-deep on their bikes. They look at you strangely but politely as they pass, tipping their head or squeaking out a faint smile. A few turn towards you in mild disbelief, contemplating your Occidentalism, shocked to see you standing at the side of their street staring into the flow. There is no aggression, just honest curiosity. Very few people travel to this devastated part of the world. A year ago it was dangerous; Western tourists were robbed and held hostage by army renegades who hadn't been paid. During the terror of Pol Pot and his Khmer Rouge, the streets of Phnom Penh were a battlefield. It is hard to spot people today in their forties and fifties gliding past on the bikes; they are all gone — murdered. People say if you grab a handful of soil in Phnom Penh, you can wring the blood out of it.

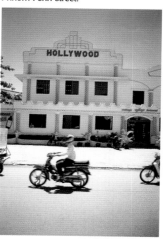

Phnom Penh street.

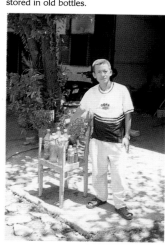

Phnom Penh gas station with gas stored in old bottles.

Darkness falls hard in the city, pushing the human-
ty away. No one is around, a few dogs sniffing bitterly
at rubbish; hoping. The only light in the street is the
bobbing, dim beam of an occasional boy on his motorbike taxi looking for an improbable fare. As he turns
the corner everything goes black again — intense
black.

A few bars are open. The light over the big snooker
tables cuts intensely out their doors into the silent
street, followed by the glassy smack of a break. Young
girls in leopard miniskirts control the games, hustling
cold beer. They speak aggressively among themselves
in their mystery language, critiquing shots that look
impossible and arguing. The balls bank back and forth,
then fall with a click into the meshed pockets. High
nasal voices squeal as the balls drop like it's child's
birthday party. Other girls who have migrated from
Vietnam sit on the sidelines wearing silky gowns, looking for "Lucky Money" as they call it. Their eyes stay
two steps ahead of the action around the bar, warm
and inviting at first then bloodthirsty and dangerous.

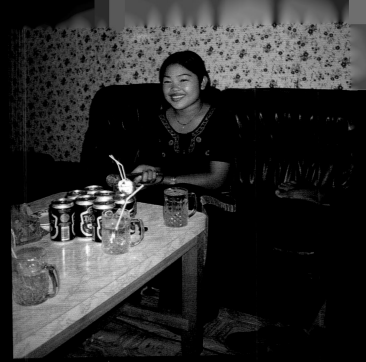

Phnom Penh Karaoke girl.

Phnom Penh bar girl.

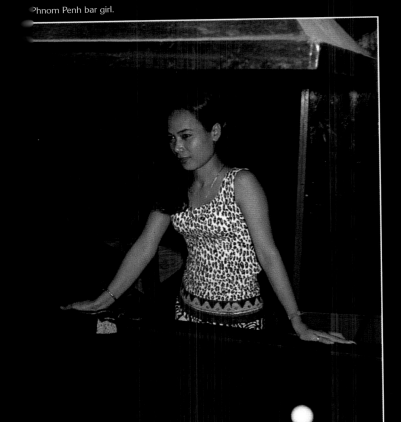

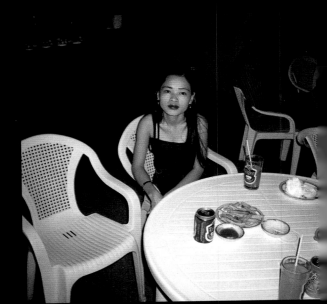

Phnom Penh bar girl.

Some streets have strange karaoke massage par-
lors hidden behind metal security gates. As you
pass, the rickety gates fly open with a screech, re-
vealing a room full of young girls sprawled across
broken down couches, wearing coordinated poly-
ester outfits. They drag themselves up and stand
like department store mannequins staring out the
door into the street. Upstairs, there are small badly
lighted rooms with gaudy, mismatched flowered

Most of the girls have tattoos tucked out of sight, traditional marks women in the sex trade wear for protection from HIV and venereal infection. They include dots under the chin or tiny Khmer letters that run in a line towards the index finger on the back of the hand. The girls explain that they do not want them to be photographed. They want no record of it, nothing that will identify them in the future as a bar girl or sex worker. This rough life is a temporary reality, something that will pass like the terror of a bad dream.

The trip from Bangkok to Phnom Penh was difficult and exhausting. An ex-British Navy guy named Richard who managed a Bangkok bar on Sukhumvit Road invited me to travel with him and a friend who was ex-Vietnam, US Army intelligence. They were going for two days to renew their Thai visas. These guys traveled hard so we left Bangkok at 2 A.M. and went over land by bus to Trat, then by pick-up truck through an intense lightning storm to the Cambodian boarder at Hat Lek, then by boat from Koh Kong to Sihanoukville, and truck to Phnom Penh. Richard had done the trip a few times and knew the ropes.

We reached Hat Lek at 4 in the morning. It was raining like hell, the way it does during the Southwest monsoon season. The checkpoint was closed until 7 A.M., so we milled around in the rain with a few dozen Thai farmers who were preparing to bring their food into Cambodia. There were piles of vegetables and various kinds of freshly butchered meat. Rows and rows of headless, plucked chickens propped up side down on tables with their long claw feet sticking into the rain. We got some curious looks, friendly but suspicious and protective. When the boarder opened things got intense. Cambodia is a very serious place; the army officials look at you strangely, wondering what the hell you are up to. We walked the no-man's land out of Thailand into Cambodia, passing through a lot of barbed wire surrounded tightly by soldiers with automatic weapons and the farmers carrying their stuff on their backs.

Farmer at Hat Lek.

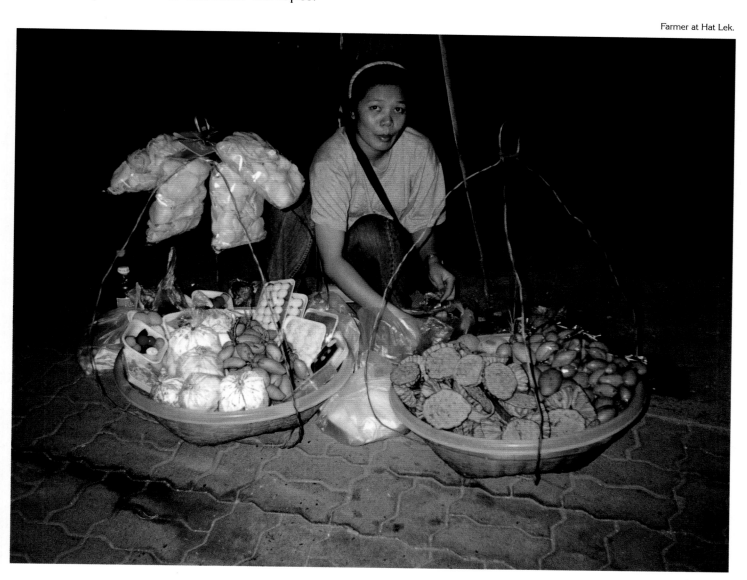

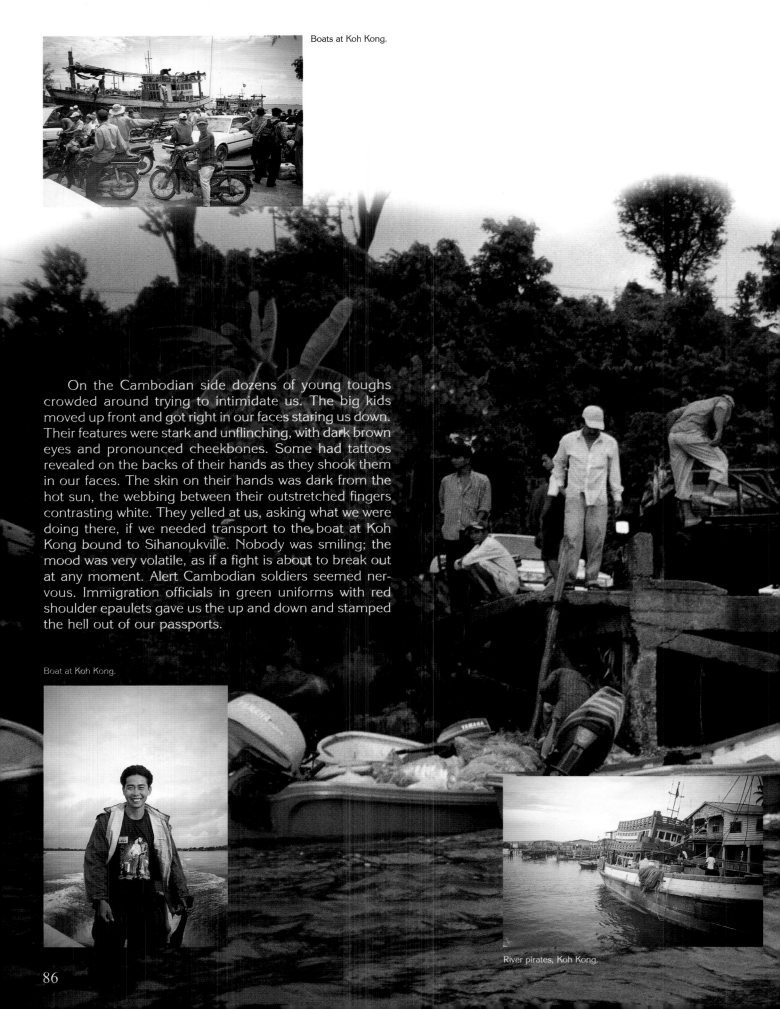

Boats at Koh Kong.

On the Cambodian side dozens of young toughs crowded around trying to intimidate us. The big kids moved up front and got right in our faces staring us down. Their features were stark and unflinching, with dark brown eyes and pronounced cheekbones. Some had tattoos revealed on the backs of their hands as they shook them in our faces. The skin on their hands was dark from the hot sun, the webbing between their outstretched fingers contrasting white. They yelled at us, asking what we were doing there, if we needed transport to the boat at Koh Kong bound to Sihanoukville. Nobody was smiling; the mood was very volatile, as if a fight is about to break out at any moment. Alert Cambodian soldiers seemed nervous. Immigration officials in green uniforms with red shoulder epaulets gave us the up and down and stamped the hell out of our passports.

Boat at Koh Kong.

River pirates, Koh Kong.

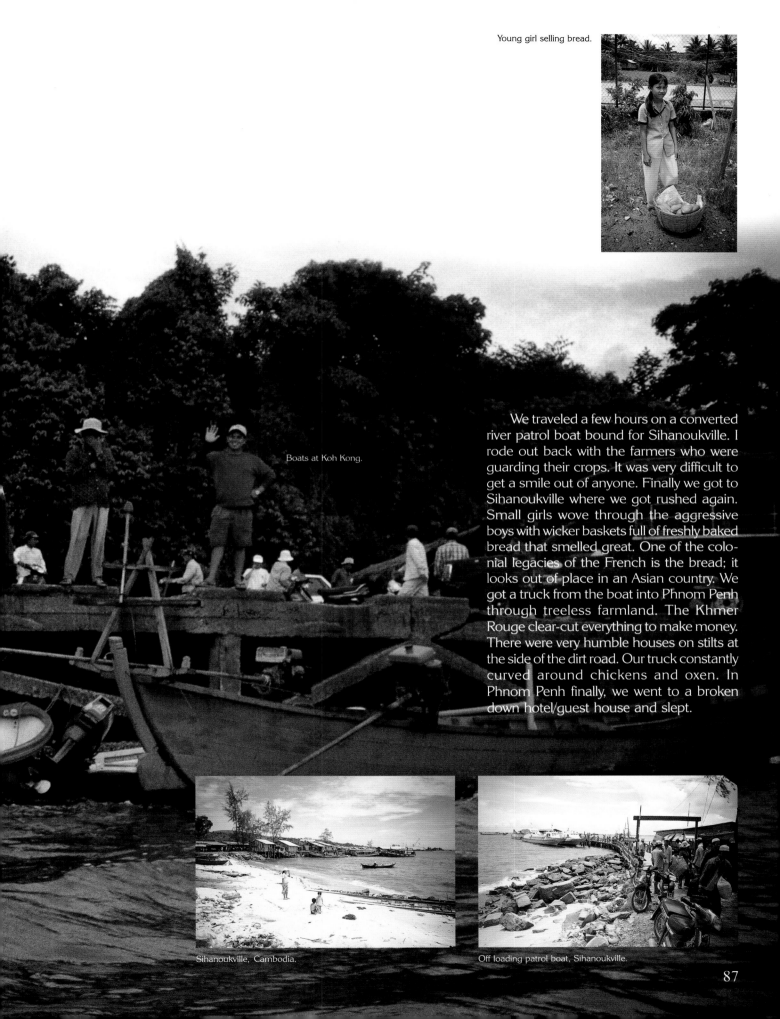

Young girl selling bread.

Boats at Koh Kong.

We traveled a few hours on a converted river patrol boat bound for Sihanoukville. I rode out back with the farmers who were guarding their crops. It was very difficult to get a smile out of anyone. Finally we got to Sihanoukville where we got rushed again. Small girls wove through the aggressive boys with wicker baskets full of freshly baked bread that smelled great. One of the colonial legacies of the French is the bread; it looks out of place in an Asian country. We got a truck from the boat into Phnom Penh through treeless farmland. The Khmer Rouge clear-cut everything to make money. There were very humble houses on stilts at the side of the dirt road. Our truck constantly curved around chickens and oxen. In Phnom Penh finally, we went to a broken down hotel/guest house and slept.

Sihanoukville, Cambodia.

Off loading patrol boat, Sihanoukville.

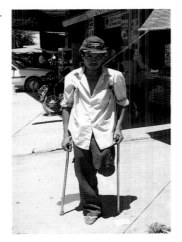
Landmine victim, Phnom Penh.

Moving around the city by driver is advised for personal safety. The streets of Phnom Penh are not in good shape. I met a young motorbike taxi kid named Chan who became my shadow. At night he brought me around the streets that were completely strange and mysterious, dark and dusty, passing by shops selling coffins. He was always at my guest house door every morning waiting. He was a good kid who apologized for his English skills, which in reality were miraculous. There are no movie theaters or ATM machines in all of Cambodia. Very little media of any kind. Chan thought he had heard of New York City and would pitch his head back and look at me when I told him about it.

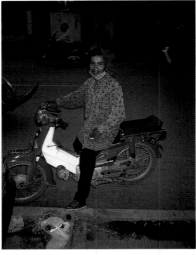

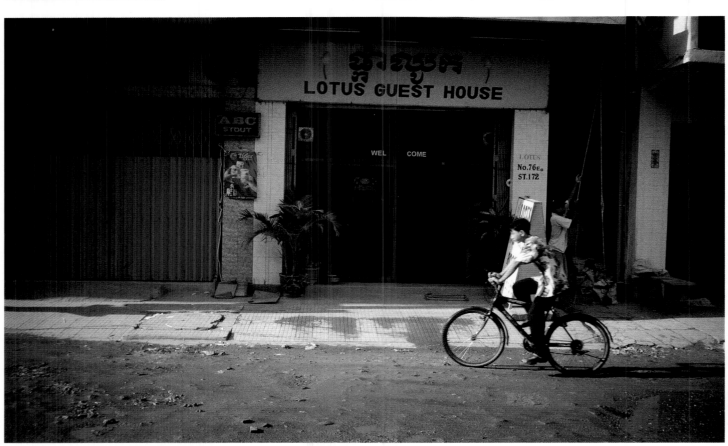
Street orphans, Phnom Penh.

Motorbike taxi driver Chan, Phnom Penh.

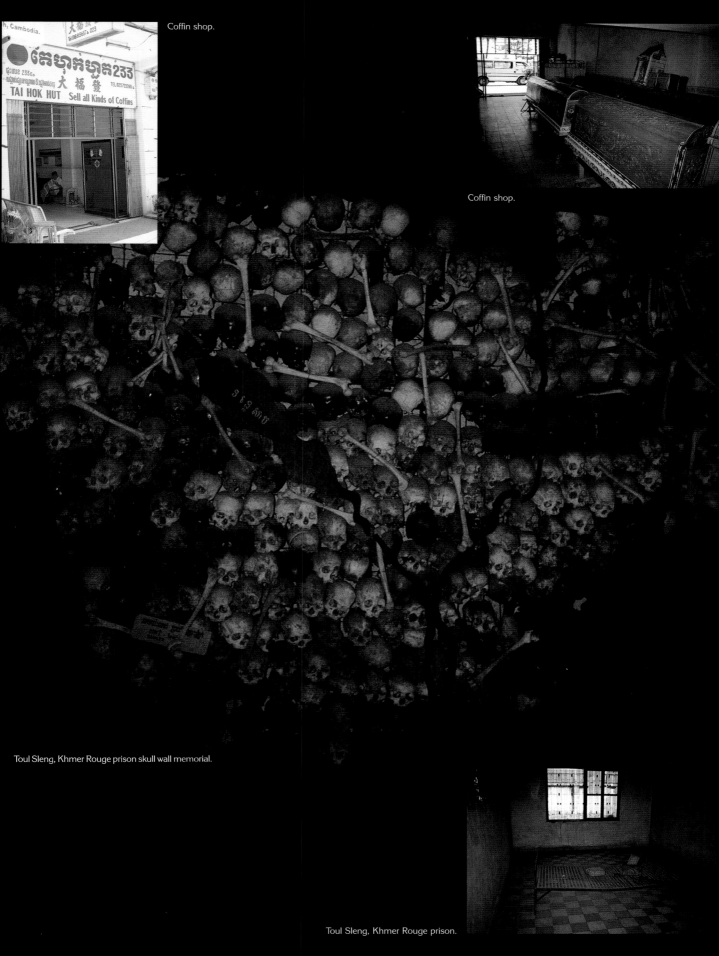

Coffin shop.

Coffin shop.

Toul Sleng, Khmer Rouge prison skull wall memorial.

Toul Sleng, Khmer Rouge prison.

One morning he offered to take me to a woman named Anna who wrote for *The Cambodian Daily*. She had recently written about a tattoo magician living in the outskirts of the city. The two-lane road from central Phnom Penh was congested with people on their motorbikes. There were no stop signs or traffic lights; everyone was taking the rules of the road into their own hands, zigzagging dangerously through each other. A thick haze of orange-colored road dust hung just above the traffic. Everyone was coughing as they rode through it.

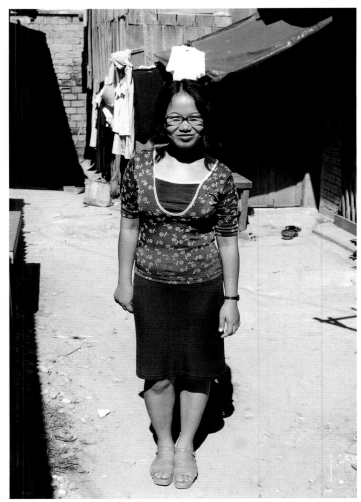

Anna from The Cambodian Daily.

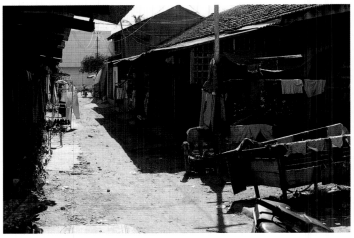

Back alley, Toul Kouk district.

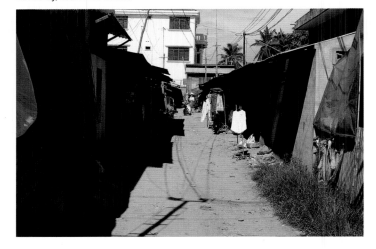

I passed through the traffic with Chan, headed to the tattoo magician's house in the Toul Kouk district. People riding next to me took note, looking surprised; they tipped their heads and smiled. Just about everyone smiled as we passed and I was amazed when I thought about the political and social chaos that these people had just gone through. I was amazed that they remembered how to smile.

The traffic slowed occasionally for large haywagons crammed with 30 young men and women on their way to factory and agricultural jobs. The slow-moving tractors that pulled the wagons moved to the side of the road when the traffic behind them built up. Most of the workers smiled big toothy, sweet smiles as we passed. They were all wearing straw hats of various styles pulled down tight.

We took a left down a narrow lane flanked with humble, thrown together shacks. Lines heavy with laundry crisscrossed between the houses, green and red plastic washtubs leaned against the walls. A few small children noticed me on the back of the motorbike and paused, staring.

90

Kong Sengheurn had a bad stomachache and could not come into the sun to speak with us about his tattooing, preferring that we come inside his shack. There was a wooden cage on the ground at the front door that had a ten-foot long python snake coiled up in it. Its tongue spit in and out nervously as I bent down for a closer look. It was dark inside Kong's house, only the light that filtered through the outside door. Space was limited, enough room for a bed, a dresser, a chair, and a table. The woven palm mat walls were neatly plastered with Hindu images of Genesha, Vishnu, and Bramha, surrounded by sacred Khmer script. People who came to be tattooed, would have to squint through the dim light to chose a design. It was oppressively hot in the front room. Kong was curled on his bed, holding his side as his small son scrambled up next to him. He pointed at his stomach shaking his head to say "No good."

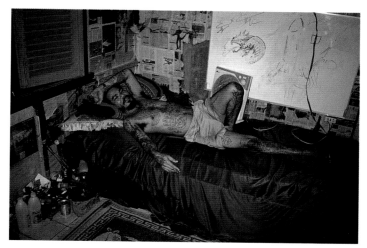

Kong Sengheurn, tattoo magician.

Kong Sengheurn.

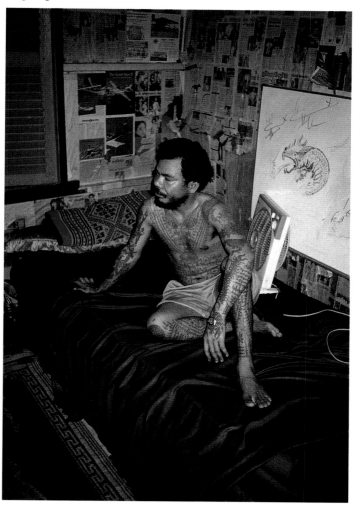

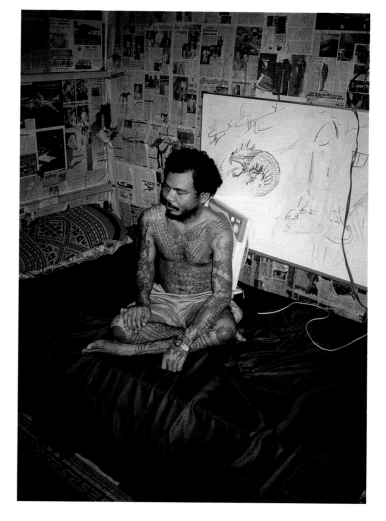

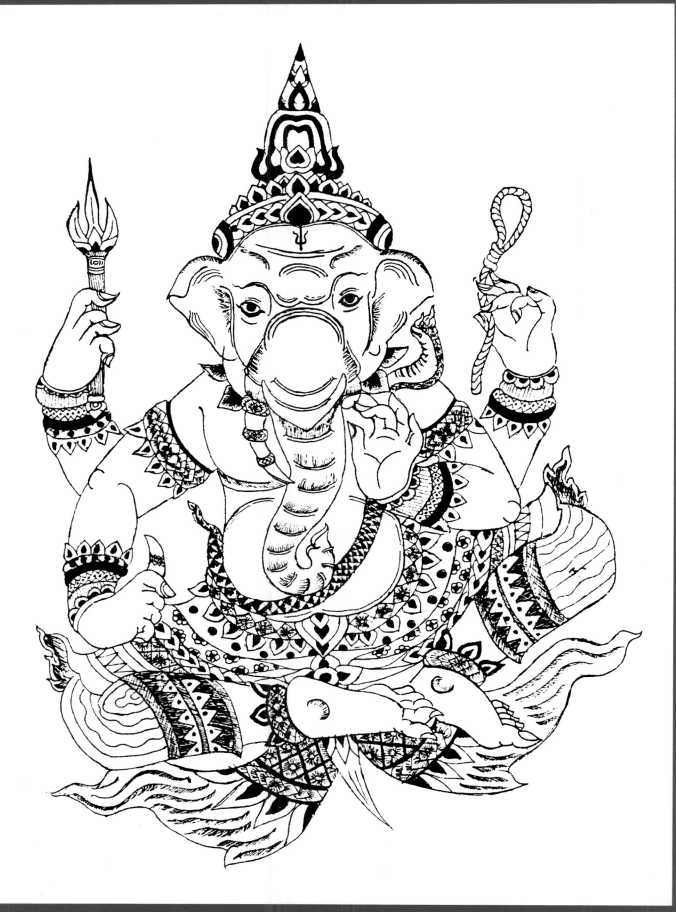

Ganesh tattoo design in Kong's house.

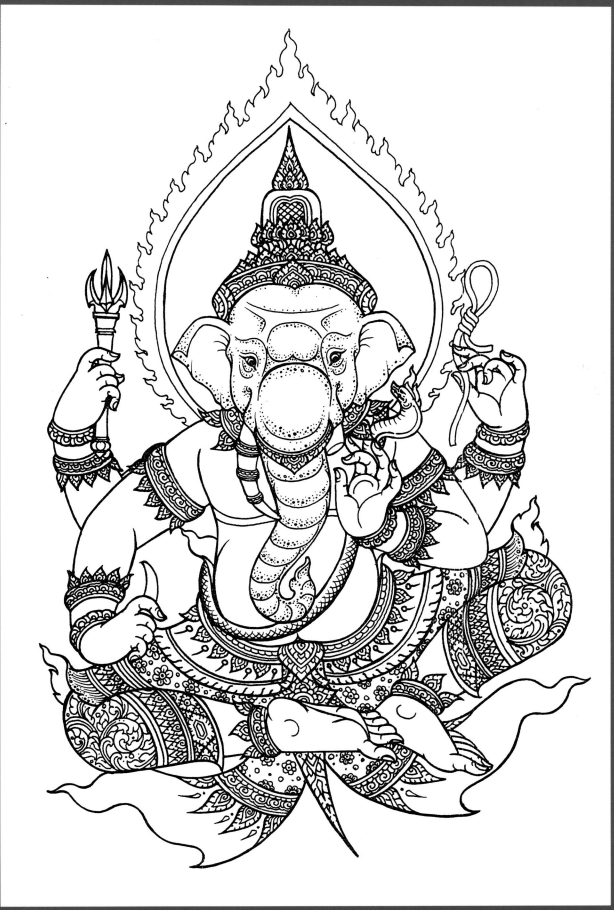

Ganesh tattoo design in Kong's house.

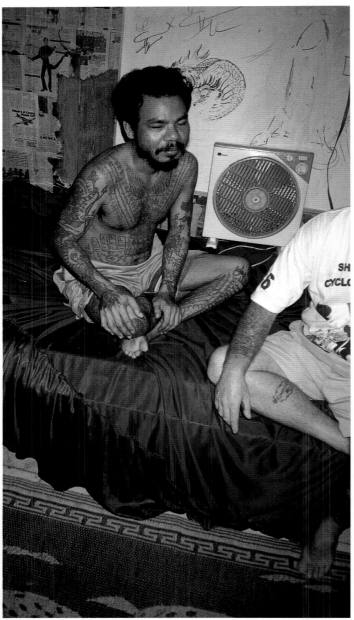

Kong Sengheurn.

Kong was a Khmer Rouge soldier at the Kao I Dang refugee camp in Thailand, where he met a monk named Uk Thuon and studied with him for four years. After the monk died, he returned to become a soldier, but now that the Khmer Rouge have largely disbanded, he tattoos outside of Phnom Penh. He is known as a Magic Man and is one of the few left who remembers the spells and traditional images. Most magic men were rounded up with Buddhist monks and killed by the Khmer Rouge during the late 1970s and early 1980s. Magic Men are known for their supernatural powers; they can kill a bull with one punch and catch bullets in their teeth. Today, young Cambodians no longer find the practice valuable. Fifty or sixty years ago, the tattoos were seen as powerful; when you were angry the images on your arms would prickle. Kong explained that his tattoos would itch with the approach of danger; the skin with the tattoos would become very bright and stand up like a frog's. His body was completely crammed, from his neck to his ankles, with Sanskrit, magical Khmer writing, and old Khaum Cambodian script surrounded with images of Hindu and Buddhist deities.

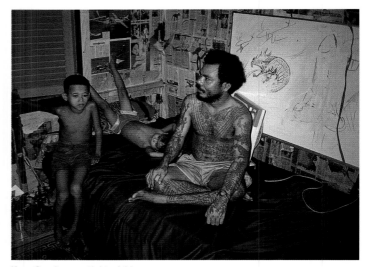

Kong Sengheurn with his children.

Kong Sengheurn's son displaying his father's tattoo machine.

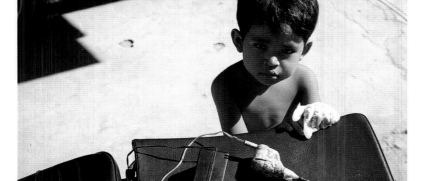

Until an Austrian tourist gave him an electric tattoo machine and modern needles two years ago, he worked by hand. Now, he doesn't care how a tattoo is applied. Cambodia is more developed than it used to be and there is sporadic electricity coming into this shack. Most Khmers prefer modern tattoos. Some continue to ask for traditional magical symbols and images but think that the old hand method is too painful.

94

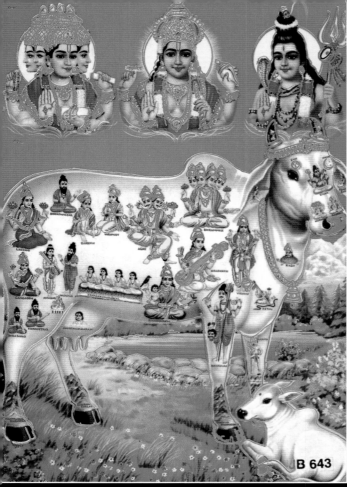

Hindu deities; Brahma (left), Vishnu (center), Shiva (right)

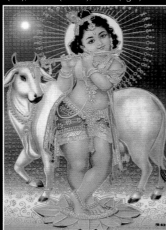

Vishnu

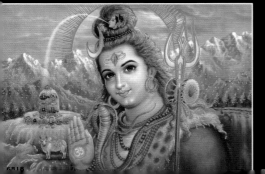

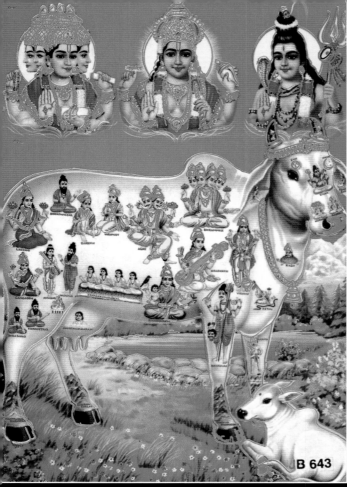

Brahma

There are a few who come to Kong to learn the traditional methods and symbolism. He asks them to prepare for the process and they should offer him fresh fruits and incense. They should also bring a large piece of cloth that will be used during the ceremony. Magic Men like Kong do not charge money for their tattoos. They tattoo people in the spirit of humanity and guidance. If there is a payment, the amount is left up to the person getting tattooed.

The tattoo images on Kong's walls of Hindu and Buddhist deities represent a process of Indianization descending through Khmer culture and filtering into other areas of Indochina since the first century A.D. At its peak, the Khmer civilization extended from its seat at Angkor to what are today Burma, northeast Thailand, and parts of Laos. Cambodia was a post along the ancient trade route between the southern kingdoms of India and China. Religious beliefs from India were first embraced by Khmer people in the southern state of Funan, which faces the Gulf of Thailand. The Khmer ruling class adopted what it could use from Indian religion and culture such as Hinduism, Buddhism, and the Sanskrit language, which introduced a writing system and the first inscriptions. Sanskrit came to be the language of the elite focussing on the deeds and merits of kings. Khmer developed as the language of the common person, focussing on daily life an inventory of material goods, land, and cattle ownership. The Hindu religious deities Brahma, Shiva and Vishnu, known as the Trinity were embraced early by the Khmer people around the fifth century and inspired religious cults that continue to be worshipped energetically today by many in Indochina.

The Khmer believe that Lord Brahma is the creator, Lord Vishnu the maintainer, and Lord Shiva the destroyer. Kong himself had the images tattooed conspicuously on his ribs, arms, and back. The multi-faced image of Lord Brahma reigns supreme for many in Indochina and it is popular for men to have him tattooed in the middle of their chest. Borrowing from Hindu thought, Khmer believe there are three modes of nature: passion is for creation, goodness is for maintenance, and ignorance is for destruction. Brahma rules the mode of passion, Vishnu the mode of goodness, and Shiva the mode of ignorance.

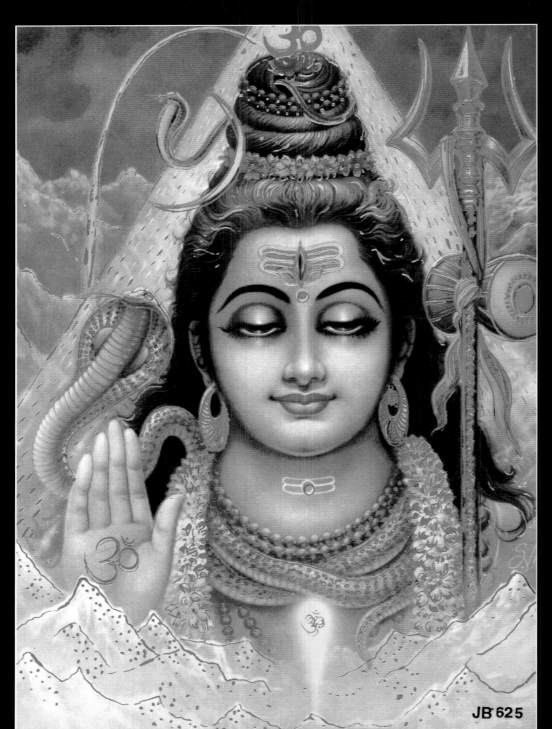

JB 625

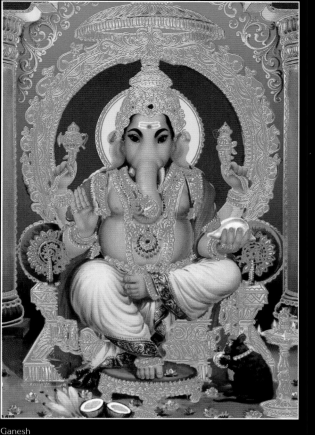

Ganesh

Secondary gods and deities are also popular tattoo motifs. Ganesh, the god of prosperity and wisdom and the deity Hanuman the Monkey King, who is Lord Rama's protector, are both used. Kong also had Buddhist images on his wall, particularly the Bodhisattva Avalokiteshvara called Lokeshvara in Cambodia, who is the image of compassion. The Mayhayana form of Buddhism was introduced to Khmer culture around the same time as Hinduism and ascended in popularity by the twelfth century. During the fourteenth century, the Theravada form of Buddhism became popular and it remains today as the fundamental faith of the people.

Hanuman the Monkey King.

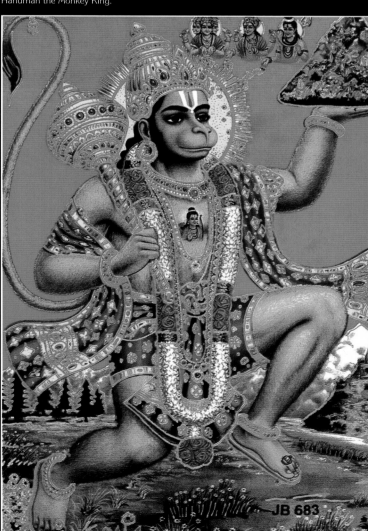

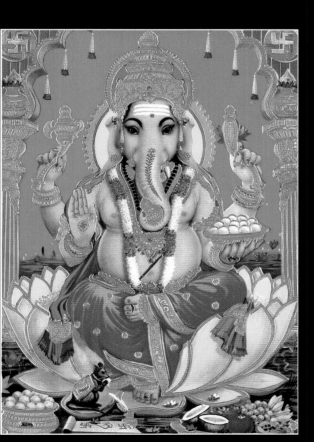

Ganesh

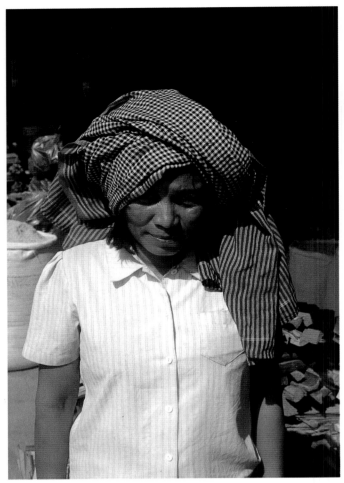
Woman laborer, Siem Reap, Cambodia.

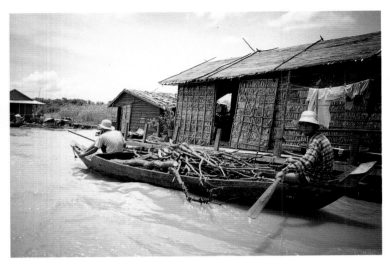
Boat carrying fire wood down Klong Yai.

The dramatic Khmer temple complex of Angkor Wat, Angkor Thom, and Ta Prohm, located outside the sleepy northern Cambodian town of Siem Reap, houses a treasury of the Khmer pantheon that has been transformed over time into the powerful tattoo lexicon of Indochina. The French naturalist Henri Mouhot, who rediscovered the overgrown jungle complex in 1861, described it saying, "At the sight of the temples, one feels annihilated beyond imagination; one looks, admires and struck with awe, remains silent."

The narrow, worn-out riverboat I took from Phnom Penh to Siem Reap coursed the 250 km up the Tonle Sap River for nearly five hours. Roughly forty men, women, and children were in the enclosed main cabin; crammed into uncomfortable, beaten-up seats. Some tried to talk over the roar of the engine, holding their noses from strong diesel fuel fumes that saturated the cabin. Fishing villages moved past outside the scratched boat windows. People wearing conical straw hats bobbed by in our wake, pramming along in little three-person, flat-bowed boats. Some larger boats had exposed, greasy engines with 10 feet long propeller shafts running back into the muddy water.

The river widened into the huge Tonle Sap Lake for more than an hour and then narrowed as the boat neared the huge hill called Phnom Krom. There were temporary fishing villages along the shore as we neared the hill; people in small boats shuttled firewood down the narrow estuary called Klong Yai. Every rainy season the lake expands for several miles up to the edge of the hill and the people dismantle their lives and migrate away. Then as the water recedes during the dry season, they return. The ground around the fishing villages smelled like old rotten fish.

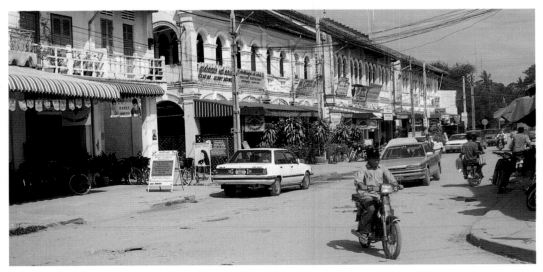
Siem Reap

The Angkor temple complex located outside Siem Reap is the largest religious monument in the world and houses the mythological images of the Khmer civilization. The roots of Indochinese tattoo iconography are inscribed on the walls of the numerous sacred and ceremonial structures. The carved reliefs at the temple locations of Angkor Wat, Angkor Thom, Ta Prohm, and Banteay Srei were created by anonymous artists between the eighth and thirteenth centuries and act as a catalog of symbols, signs, and images that reveal a framework of cultural belief. They were once thought to be completely decorative, but now are believed to be encoded texts that contain important Angkorean religious, mythological, historical, and moral concepts. Most likely, the galleries of carved images and illustrated epic texts were reserved for the eyes of the Angkorean elite. The messages of the reliefs would have been incomprehensible to the common person. Many believe that specialist priests were used to help translate the significance of the images.

Siem Reap

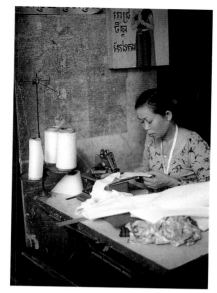

Seamstress, Siem Reap.

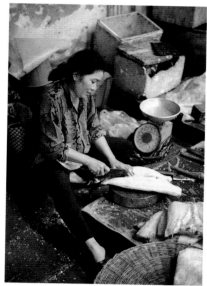

Butcher, Siem Reap.

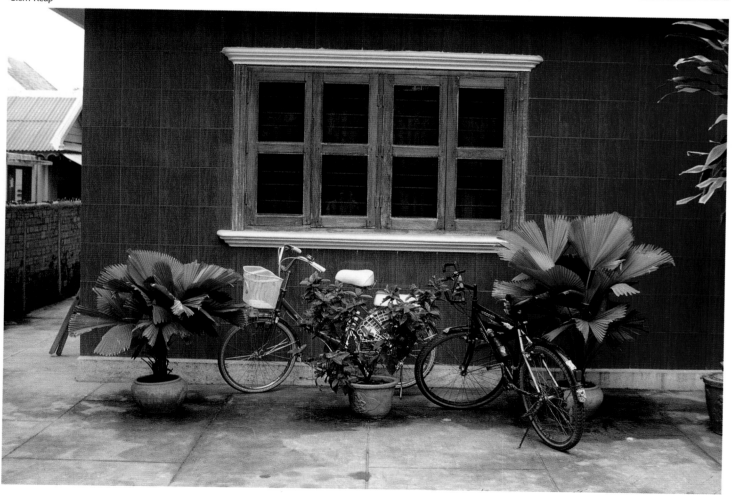

Angkor Wat Cambodia.

Angkor Wat, Cambodia.

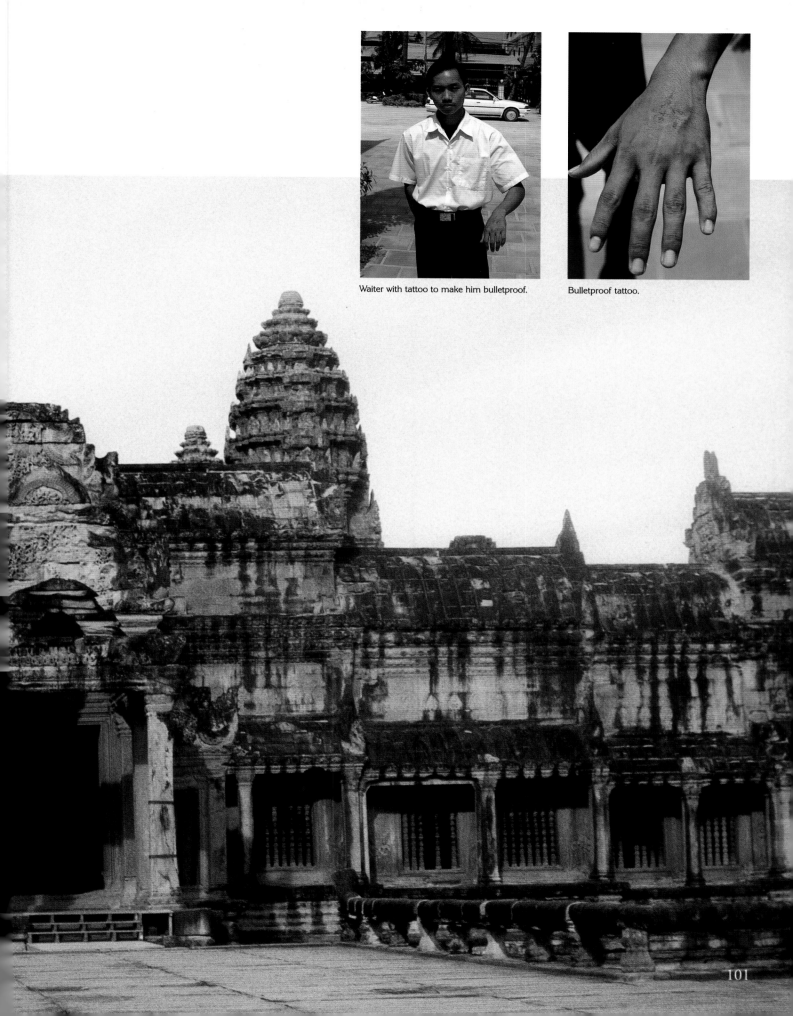

Waiter with tattoo to make him bulletproof.

Bulletproof tattoo.

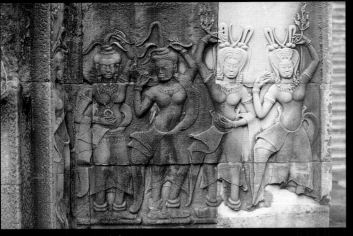

Apsara celestial dancers, relief carving.

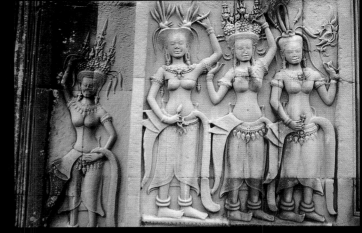

Apsara celestial dancers, relief carvings.

The stone reliefs are now seen as having an evocative and animating purpose that brought the temples to life. The carved images contributed to the realization on earth of the divine world. For example, the images on the walls of Angkor Wat narrate the history of the divine Khmer King Suryavarman II (1113 A.D.) The images on the walls of the temple Bayon illustrate the life of the Khmer King Jayavarman VII (1181 A.D.). Experts believe the images were carved in exacting detail or they would have failed in their purpose, much like powerful magical spells that are rendered useless by the omission of an important component. Angkor Wat was a funereal temple dedicated to the Hindu deity Vishnu. Banteay Srei, located just outside the complex and its incredible rose-colored sandstone carvings was dedicated to the Hindu deity Shiva. Combined, all the buildings of Angkor represent the Hindu and Buddhist universe.

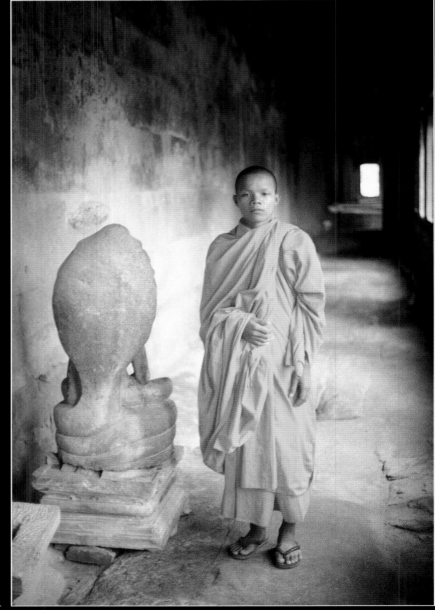

Buddhist monk in Angkor Wat.

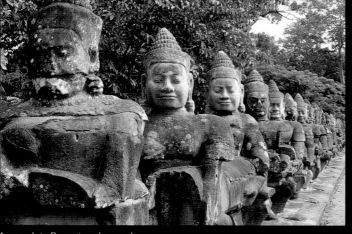
Approach to Bayon temple complex.

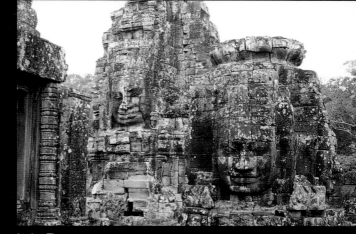
Angkor Thom.

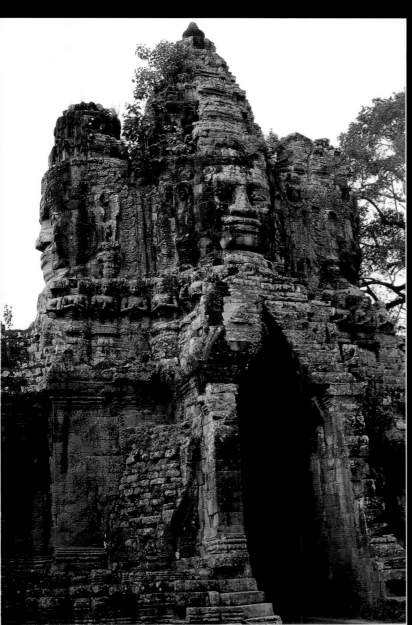
Gate at Angkor Thom.

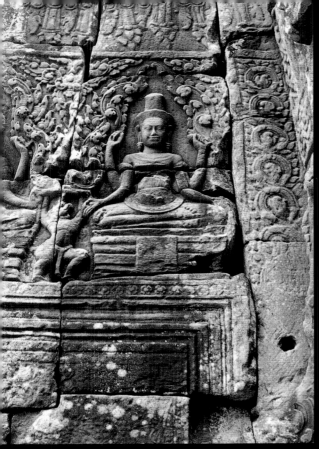

Vishnu relief carving.

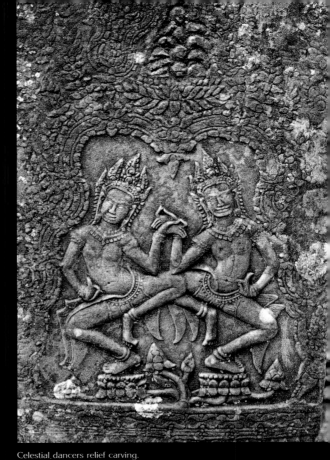

Celestial dancers relief carving.

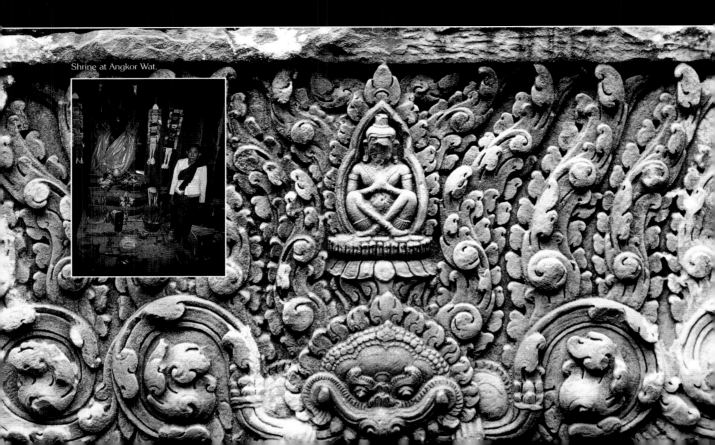

Shrine at Angkor Wat.

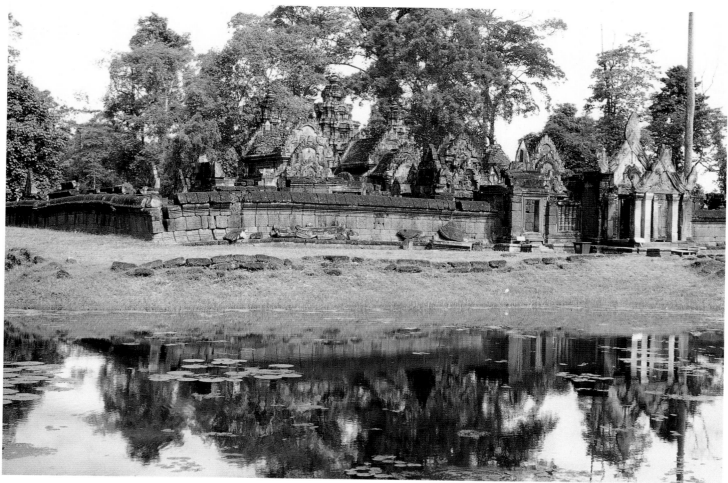
Banteay Srei temple.

As I climbed through the mysterious stone buildings, images of Shiva, Vishnu, Brahma, and Ganesh came to life just as they had on the woven mat walls at Kong's humble tattoo shack. Adolescent and teenaged Cambodian children played in the darkened monumental hallways next to sculptures that were more than one thousand years old, their cries echoing off the cool stone. Cambodian authorities dressed in blue cotton uniforms strolled gently through the remains of their early civilization, keeping tabs on the kids and visitors. Holy men and women sat next to decorative shrines of burning candles, string, and fabric they had constructed around large stone deities. Young women with their heads wrapped and protected from the hot sun poked sharp gardening tools into the crevices between the huge stones, clearing away the relentless creep of the jungle.

Girls on their way to school.

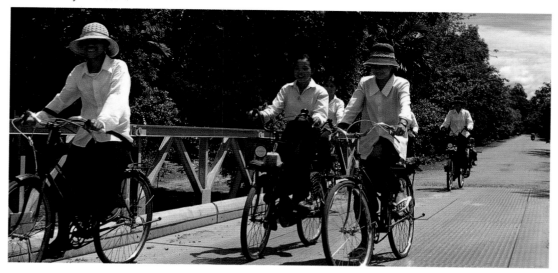

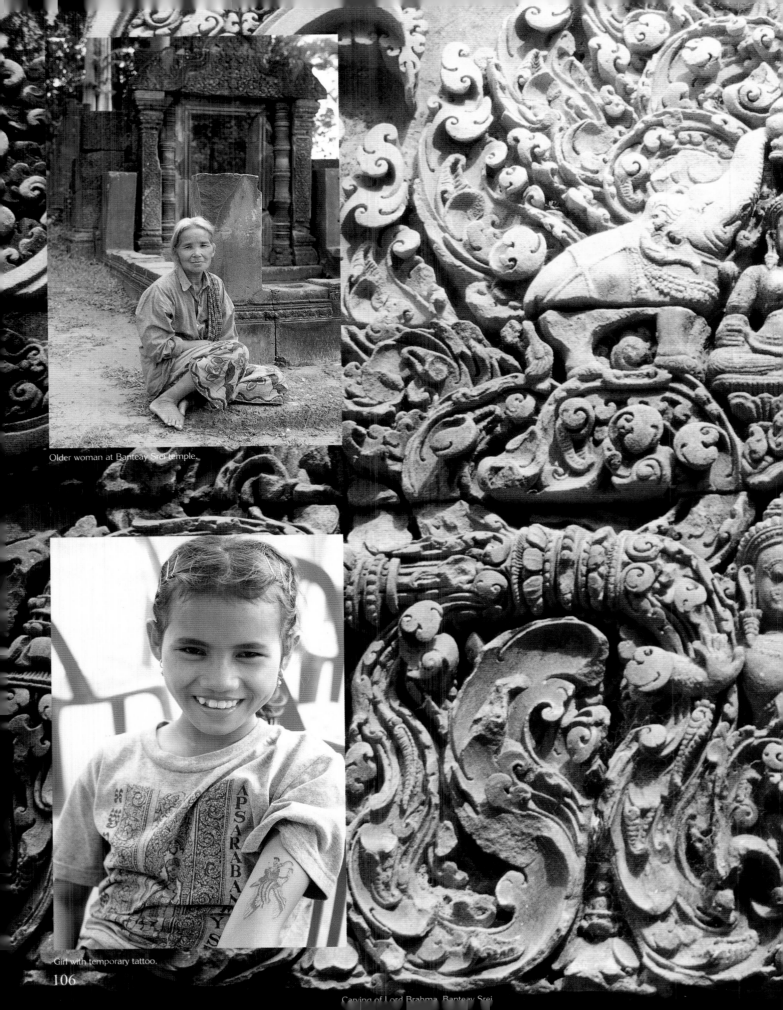

Older woman at Banteay Srei temple.

Girl with temporary tattoo.

106

Carving of Lord Brahma, Banteay Srei.

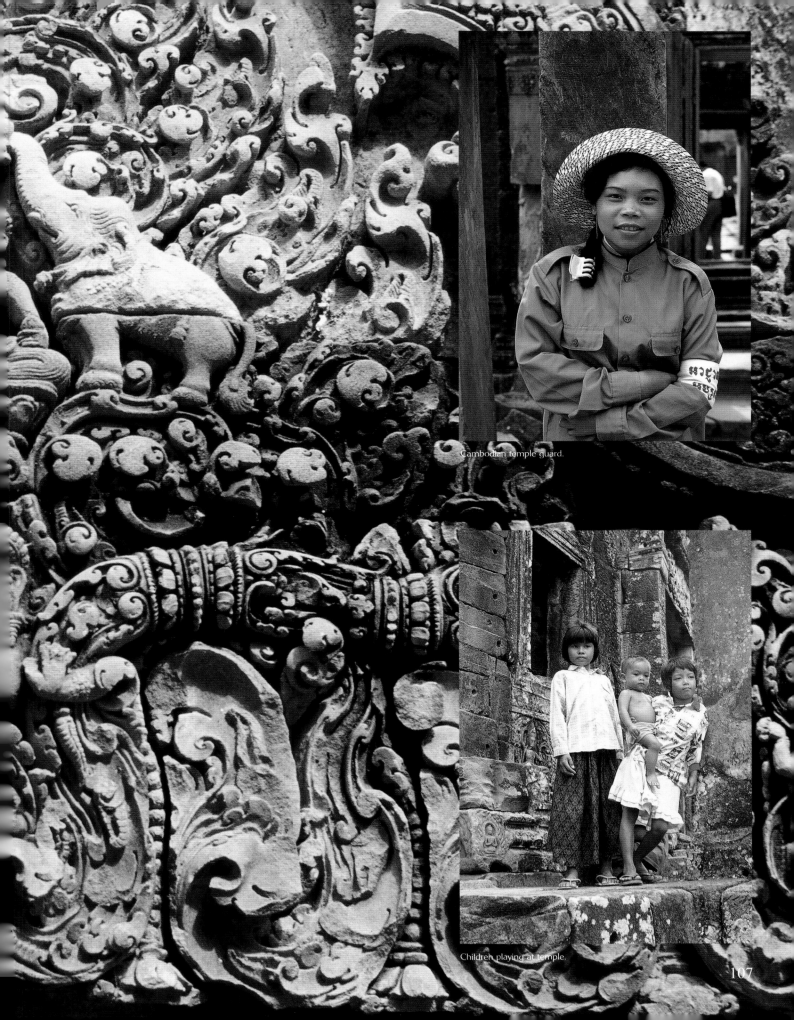

Cambodian temple guard.

Children playing at temple.

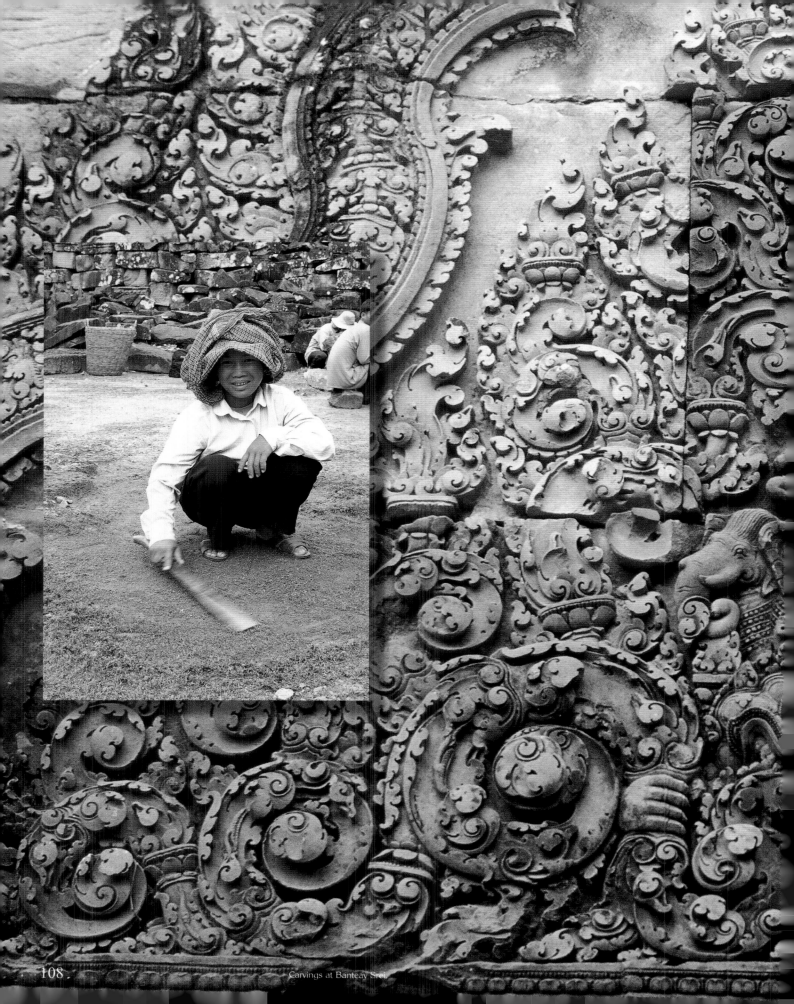

Carvings at Banteay Srei

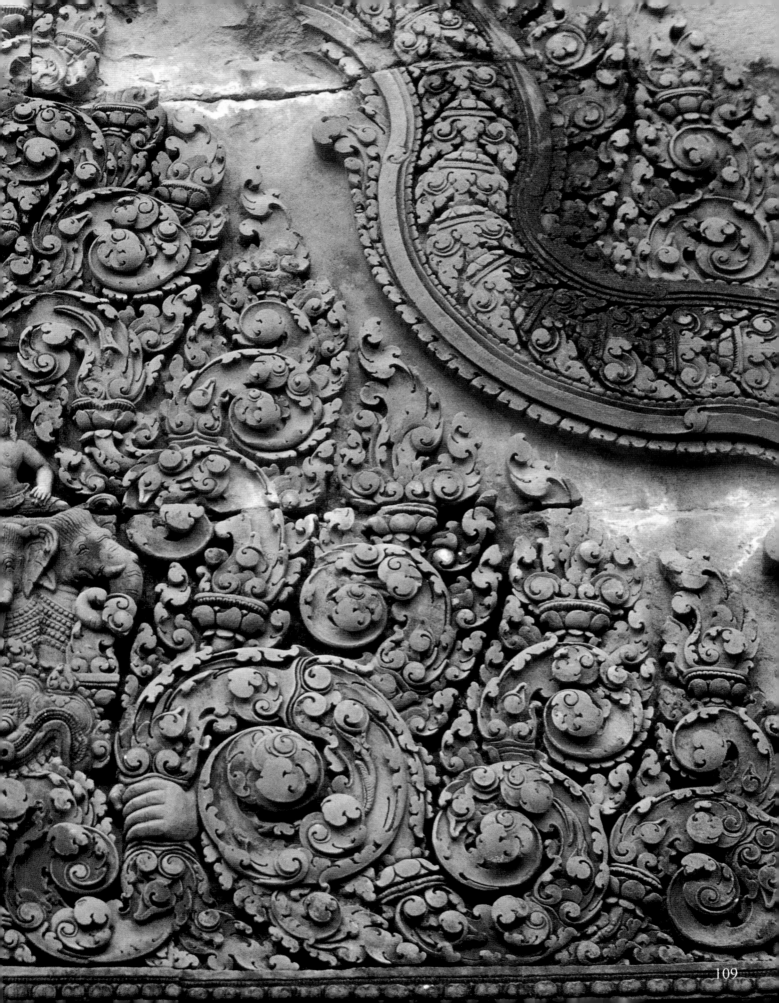

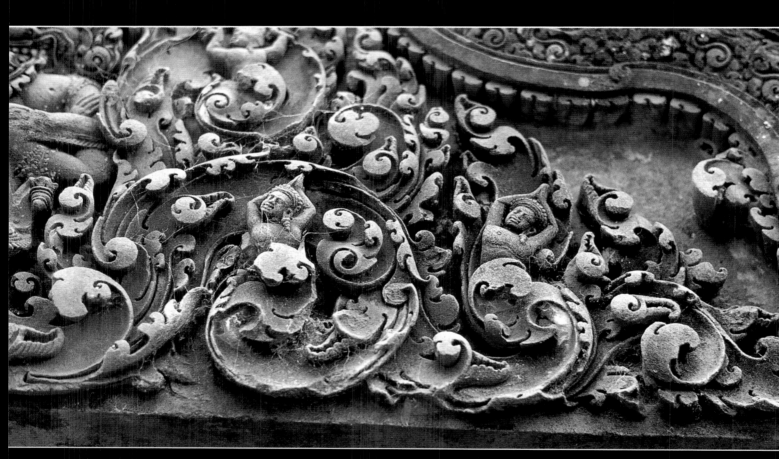

Carvings at Banteay Srei.

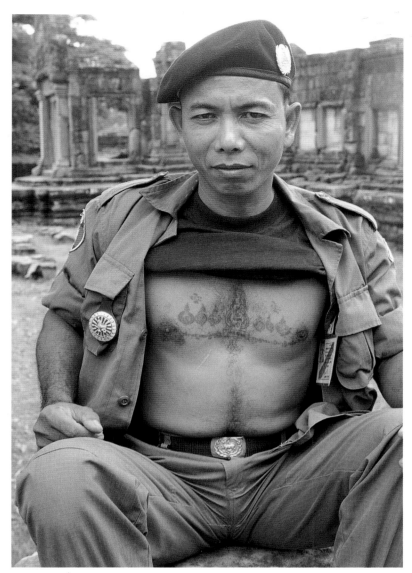

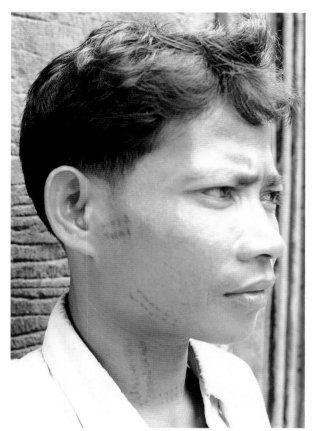

Ex-Khmer Rouge soldier with facial tattoos to ensure death if he is shot.

Ex-Khmer Rouge soldier with tattoos at his temple area to ensure death if he is shot.

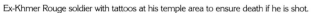

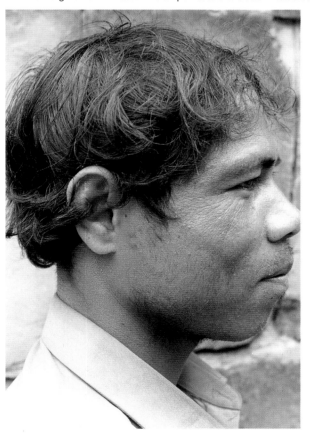

Ex-Khmer Rouge soldier with magical-animist tattoos on his chest to make him bulletproof.

Middle-aged men wearing worn military uniforms who had fallen prey to a landmine stood one-legged, propped up on crutches, leaning against walls. They smiled calmly pointing at their stump, asking for a donation. These men had most likely been members of the Khmer Rouge during the chaos of the 1970s and early 1980s. Many had prominent boxlike tattoos decorating their faces, arms and torsos. They put a box over their hearts with Khmer writing that hailed Buddha, asking that in the event they were shot, they'd get it right in the heart for a fast painless death. Others had diamond shapes tattooed across their chests or down their jaw lines. A few had blue-black diamonds above the bridge of their noses asking that if they were shot, they'd get it right between the eyes. The black diamond shapes are based more in animist superstitious belief than Buddhist faith. Some soldiers in Cambodia today continue to tattoo magical boxes over their knees, asking not to be shot there, disabled and left in the jungle to be devoured by wild animals or ants. The most feared death for a jungle soldier is to be eaten alive by ants.

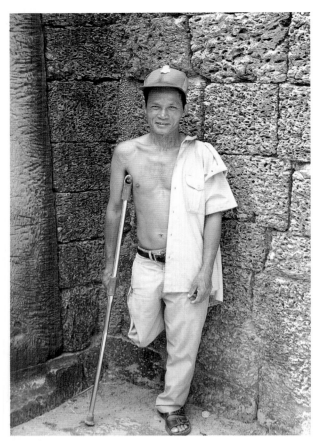

Ex-Khmer Rouge soldier, land mine victim.

Magical-animist tattoos on chest to make him bulletproof. Boxes tattooed at joints to prevent arms from being blown off in battle.

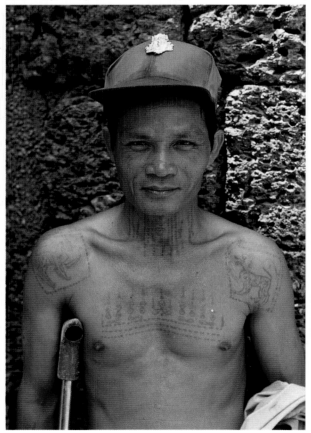

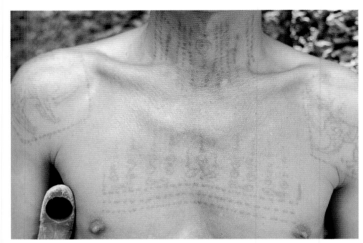

Close-up of magical tattoos.

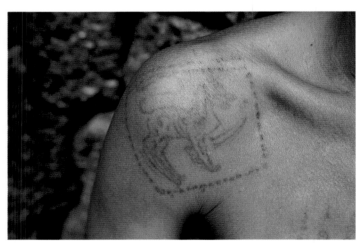

Close-up of box tattoos.

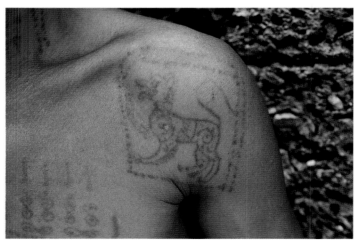

Close-up of box tattoos.

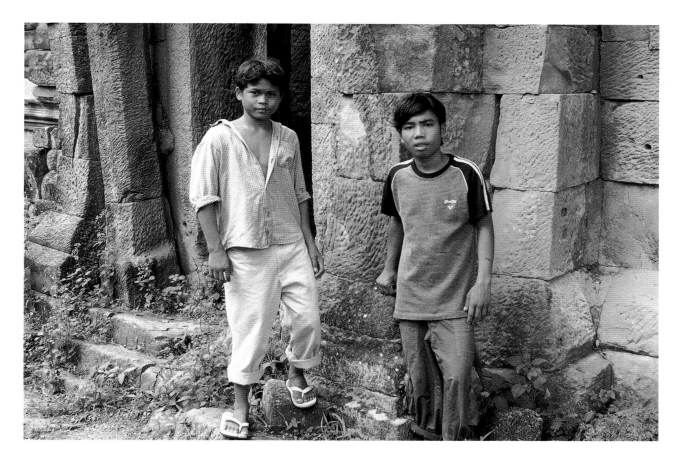

Tattooed man at Banteay Srei.

Scorpion tattoo received in Cambodian prison.

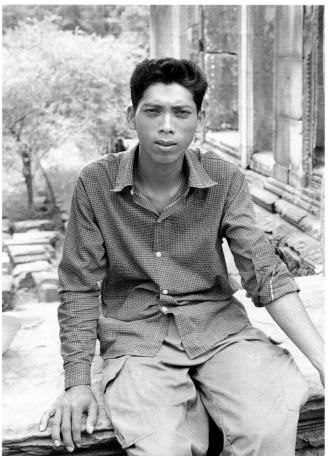

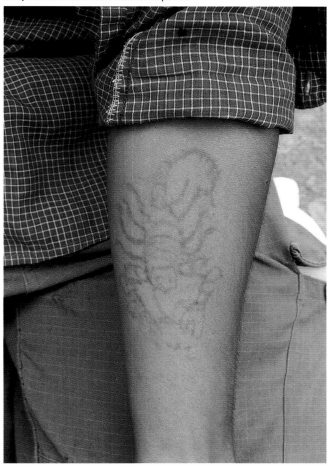

At the overgrown rear of the complex near the Terrace of the Leper King, two young boys attached themselves to me as informal tour guides. They offered to bring me into the jungle to a small Buddhist school where the monk tattooed. Both boys assured me that the presence of land mines was minimal but instructed me to walk exactly in their steps. We passed through tall trees with thick waist-high vegetation and emerged into a clearing around the humble temple school called Bria Branom. The boys introduced me to the thin, middle-aged monk named Mut who was hunched over the front porch of a temple outbuilding surrounded by his students. He had several Buddhist tattoos on his chest and back and was in the middle of drawing a protective amulet cloth for a soldier. His hand pulled a common, black magic marker over the cloth creating a design of leaping tigers surrounded with magical Khmer script. He told me through the boy's translation that magical cloths were popular among soldiers for protection from being killed. They carefully folded them up and put them in their helmets before going on patrol or into battle.

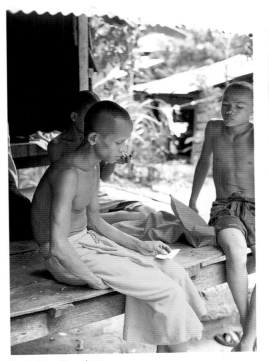

Monk Mut with students.

Jungle temple school, Bria Branom.

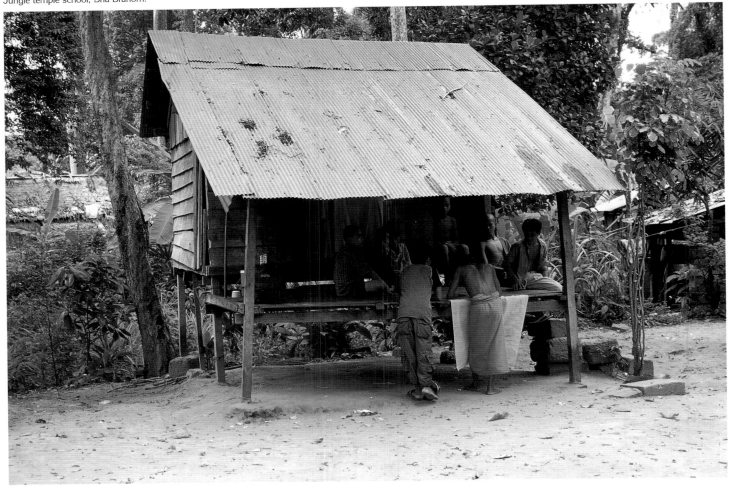

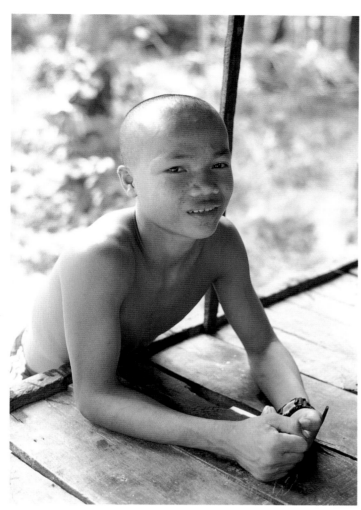

Young student at temple Bria Branom.

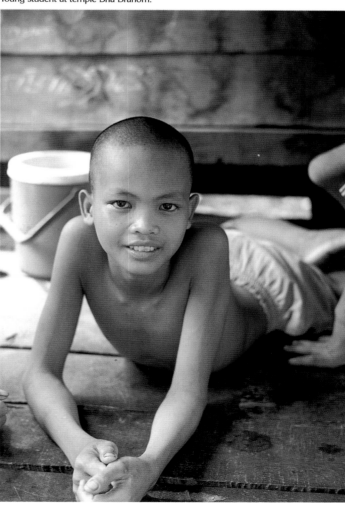

Young student at temple Bria Branom.

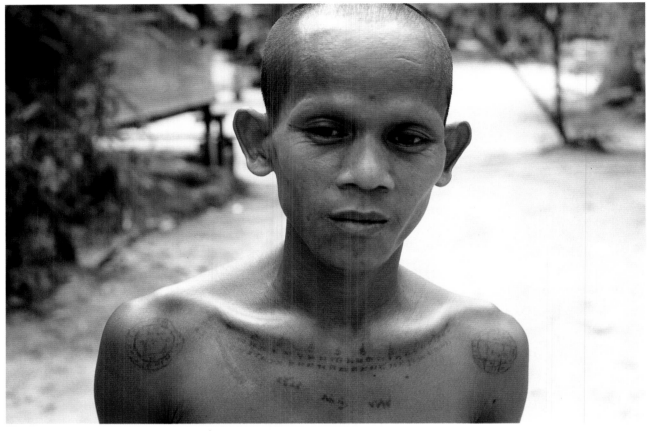

Monk Mut.

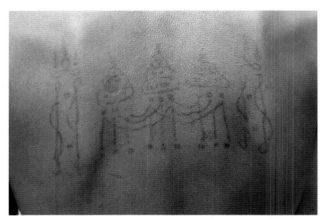

Monk Mut's back.

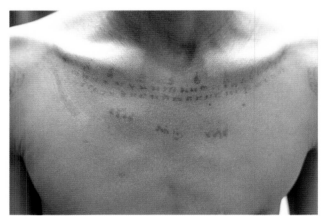

Monk Mut's chest.

116

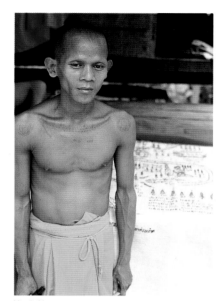
Monk Mut.

My guides suggested that I return to the monument area, they were nervous the authorities would come looking for us. As we walked back through the jungle, a middle-aged man on a motorbike wearing a plain beige button down shirt came up behind us as if he had been looking for us. The boys looked nervously at him as he stopped ten feet away. They explained he had been following us at a distance all afternoon and was there to ensure my safety. Cambodia is in dire need of the hard currency Westerners bring and in no mood for a kidnapping or killing. The man on the motorbike was my insurance policy. As he looked away momentarily, the boys pointed at the temple structures in front of us, shook my hand, and disappeared into the jungle.

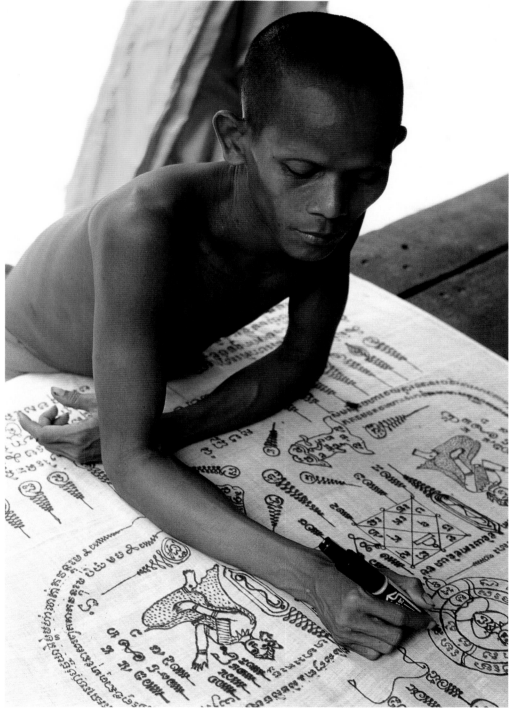
Monk Mut drawing magical cloth.

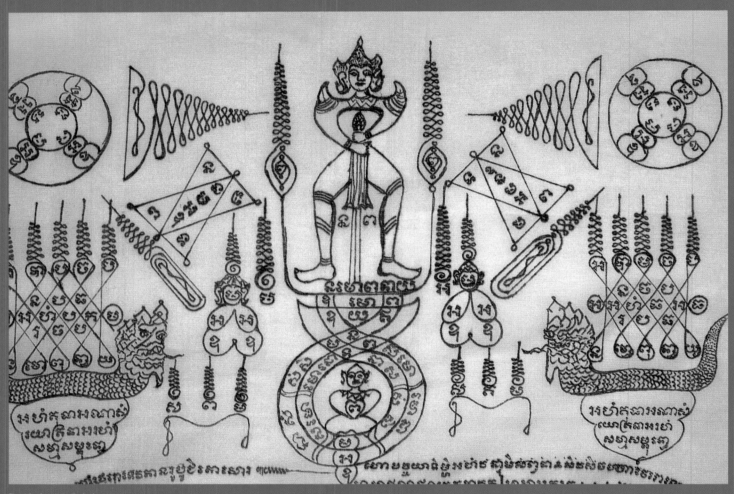

Detail of magical cloth.

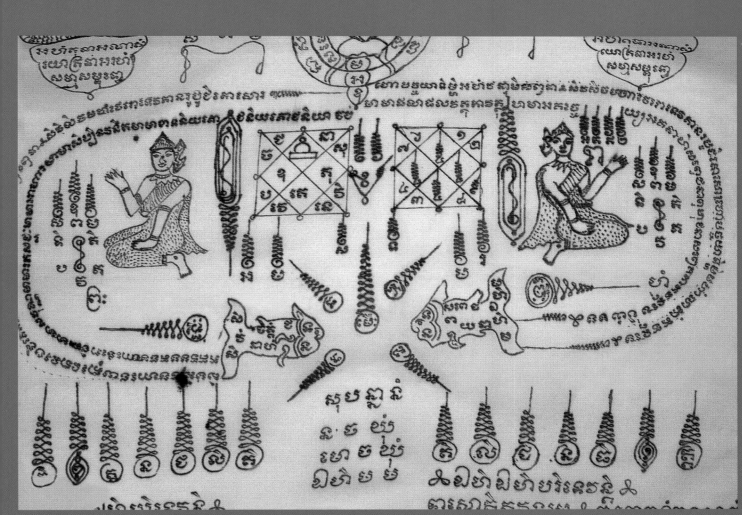

Detail of magical cloth.

Chapter Seven

Faith Power and Forgiveness

The Tattoos of Laos

The Tuk-Tuk taxi men of Vientiane, Laos, cluster in front of the sparse hotels and guest houses killing time. They sit at sidewalk tables casually playing checkers, smoking bitter smelling cigarettes, and drinking rich black coffee from steaming glasses with sweet condensed milk settled on the bottom. Most of the men are tattooed with Thom and Pali letters that decorate their wrists and arms. They are all Buddhist and animist symbols meant to prevent them from being shot, stabbed, or cut, and I wonder why. Life in the small capital City is very slow and uncongested, reflecting the overall tone of the culture and people. Laotian people are very gentle; they speak so softly you are forced to bend near as if hard of hearing.

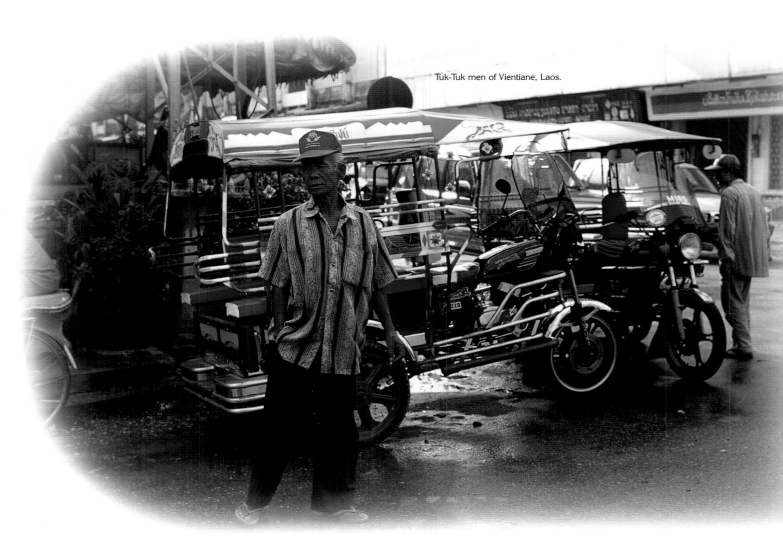

Tuk-Tuk men of Vientiane, Laos.

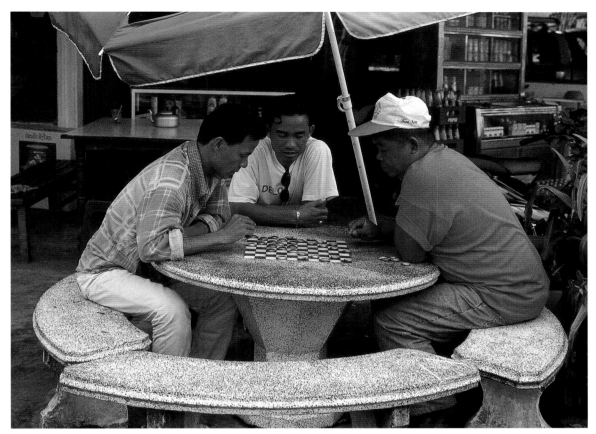

Tuk-Tuk men of Vientiane, Laos.

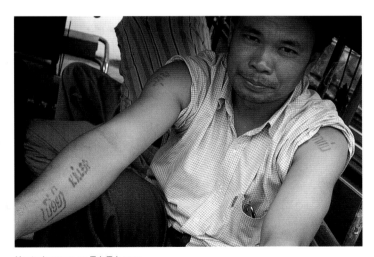

Magical tattoos on Tuk-Tuk man.

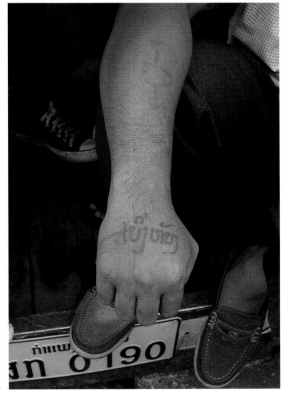

Magical tattoos on Tuk-Tuk man.

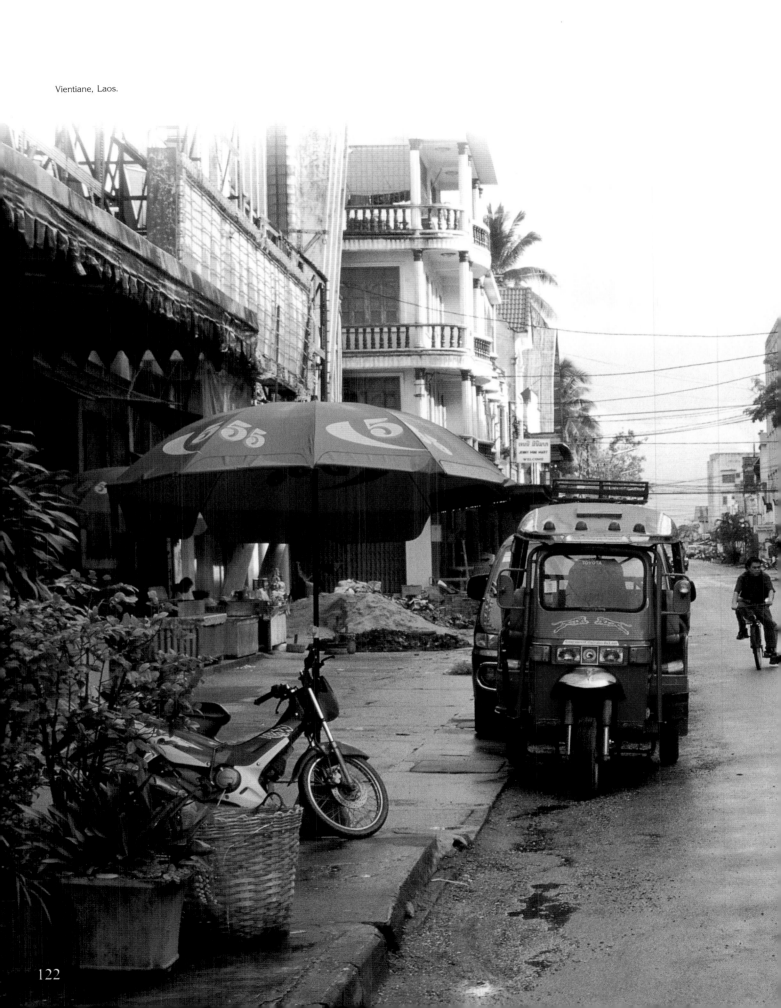

Vientiane, Laos.

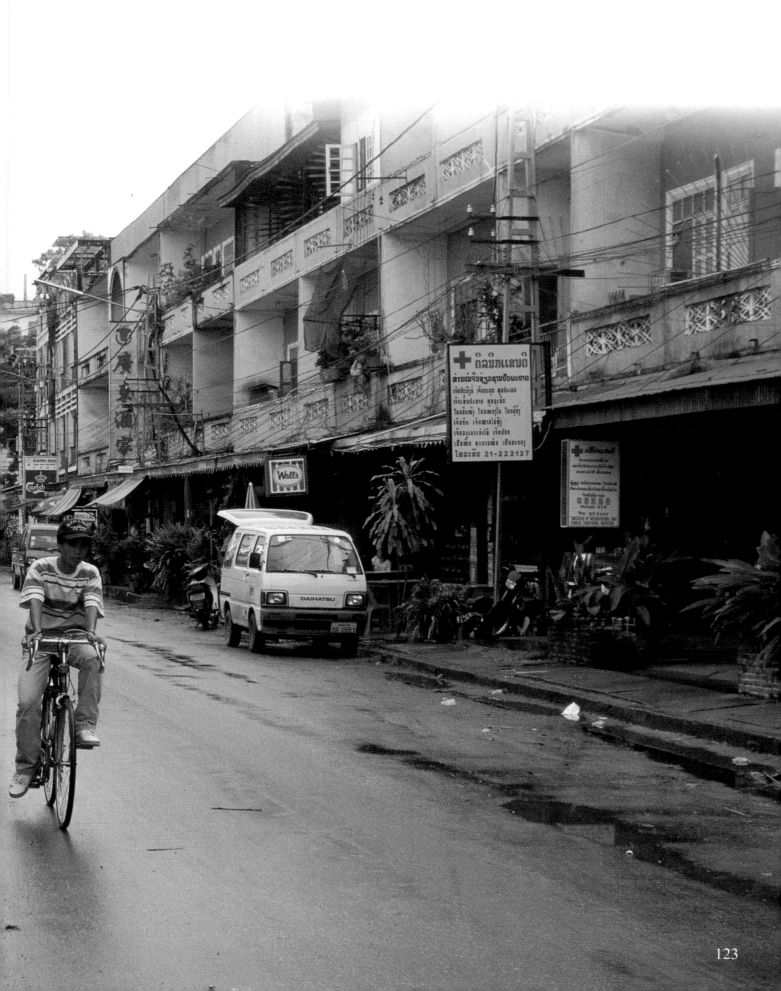

One driver named Nith looks from behind a pair of teardrop sunglasses that are slightly crooked. He puffs vigorously at his cigarette and finally exhales a huge plume of smoke that swirls around his sun darkened face. The inside of his left arm has large, crudely tattooed letters scrolling from elbow to wrist that spell out the word INTERNATIONAL. The ideological tattoo is a tribute to the coming of the Communist International, when the entire world will be united under communism. The partially reformed communist regime of the Lao People's Demo-

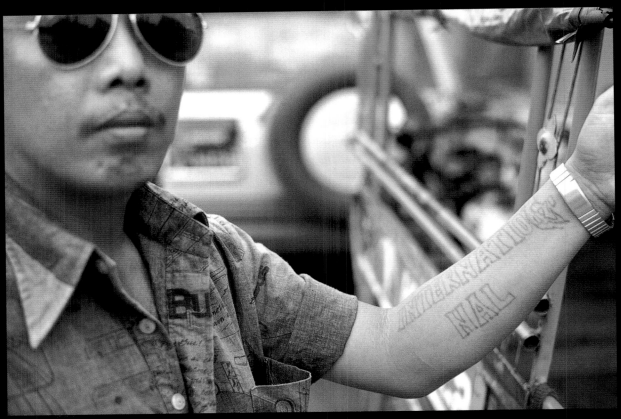

Nith with International tattoo.

cratic Republic has been in power for 25 years since the end of the Vietnam War. Nith is able to work for himself as a Tuk-Tuk driver, but the government is wary of Westerners and the outside culture they bring into the country. A middle-aged man who sees that I am talking with the Tuk-Tuk men, approaches from across the street and introduces himself in near perfect English. He is dressed in slacks and a casual button down shirt like the Tuk-Tuk men, but has possibly joined us with a different purpose in mind: to keep an eye on me.

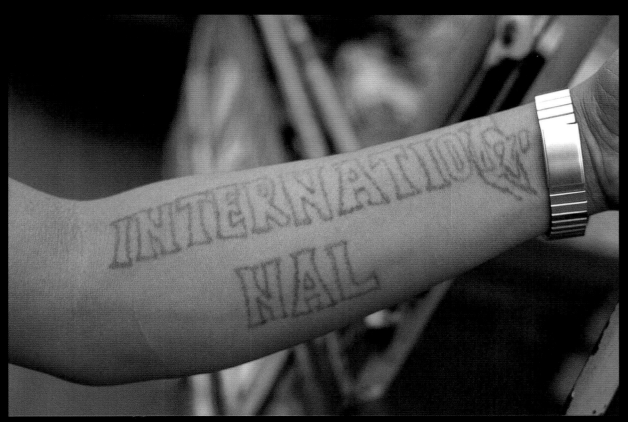

Nith's International tattoo.

Rice cultivation outside Vientiane, Laos.

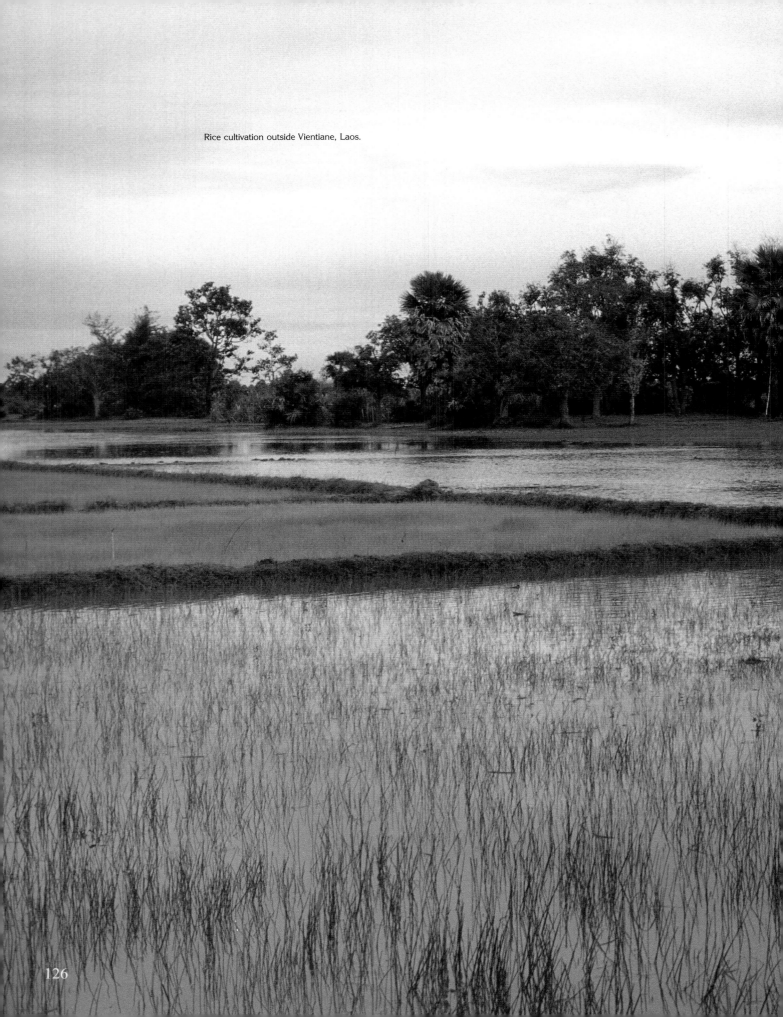

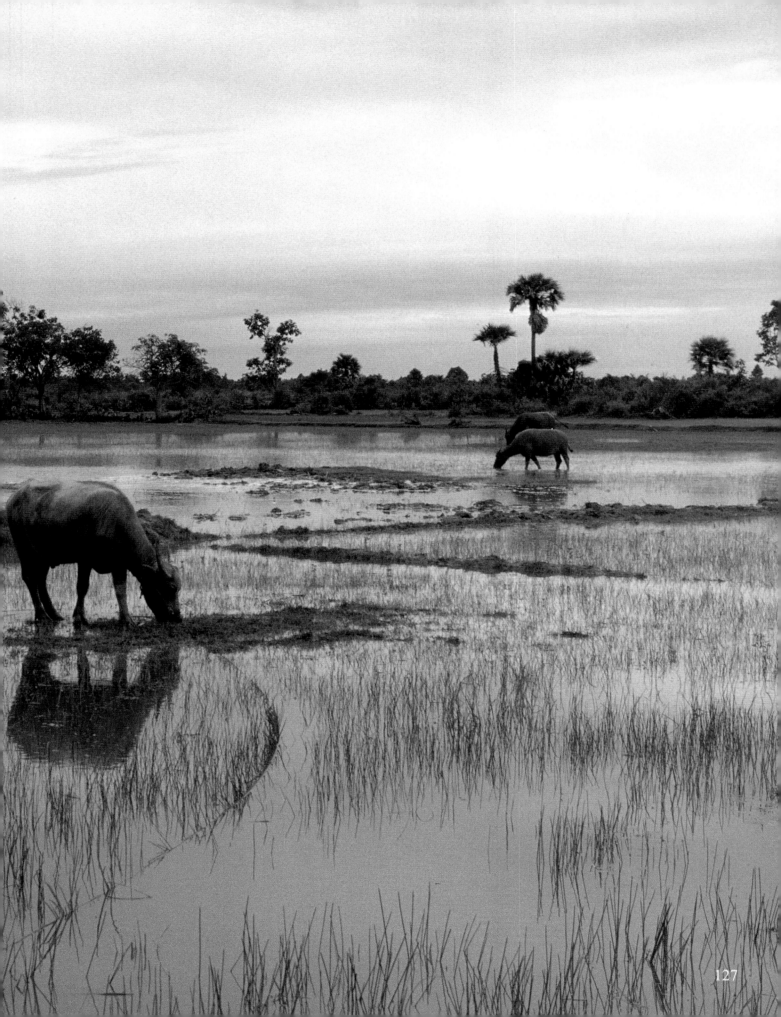

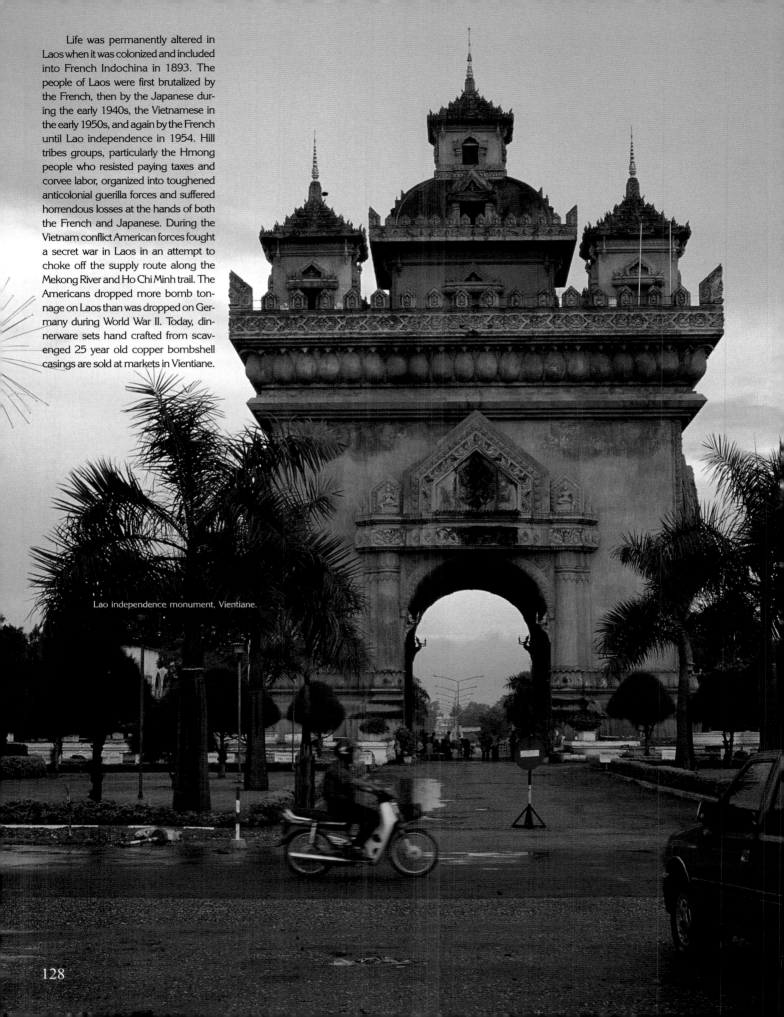

Life was permanently altered in Laos when it was colonized and included into French Indochina in 1893. The people of Laos were first brutalized by the French, then by the Japanese during the early 1940s, the Vietnamese in the early 1950s, and again by the French until Lao independence in 1954. Hill tribes groups, particularly the Hmong people who resisted paying taxes and corvee labor, organized into toughened anticolonial guerilla forces and suffered horrendous losses at the hands of both the French and Japanese. During the Vietnam conflict American forces fought a secret war in Laos in an attempt to choke off the supply route along the Mekong River and Ho Chi Minh trail. The Americans dropped more bomb tonnage on Laos than was dropped on Germany during World War II. Today, dinnerware sets hand crafted from scavenged 25 year old copper bombshell casings are sold at markets in Vientiane.

Lao independence monument, Vientiane.

128

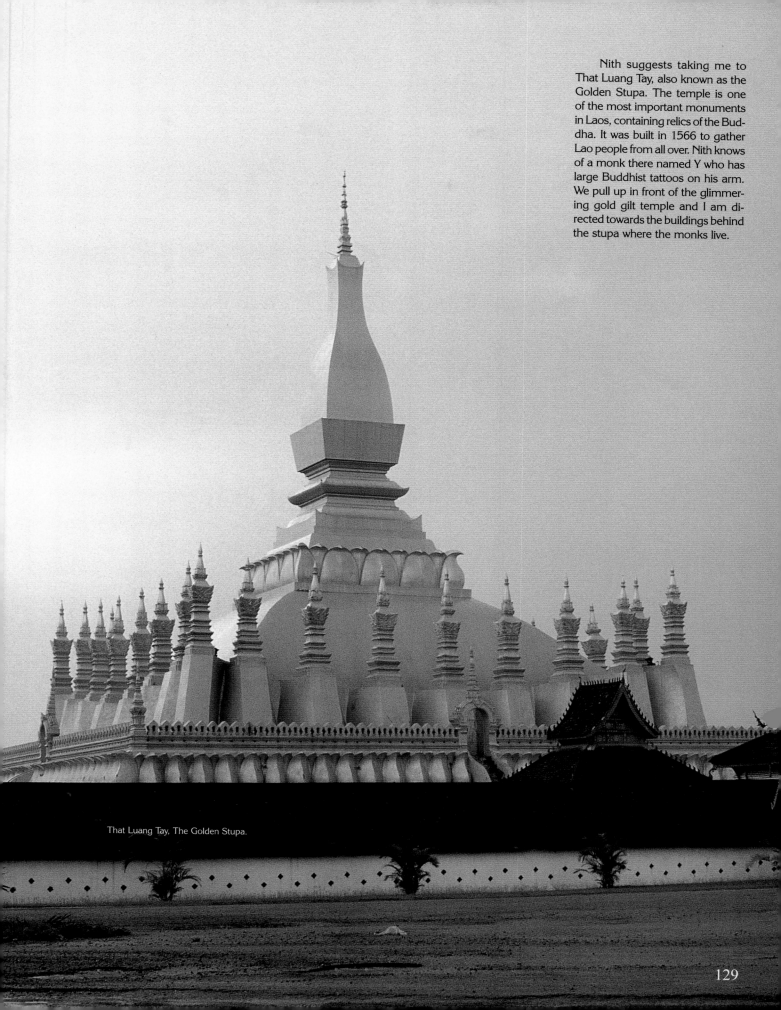

Nith suggests taking me to That Luang Tay, also known as the Golden Stupa. The temple is one of the most important monuments in Laos, containing relics of the Buddha. It was built in 1566 to gather Lao people from all over. Nith knows of a monk there named Y who has large Buddhist tattoos on his arm. We pull up in front of the glimmering gold gilt temple and I am directed towards the buildings behind the stupa where the monks live.

That Luang Tay, The Golden Stupa.

Y is sitting on the second floor balcony of his living quarters, looking out towards the stupa; drinking a glass of water in the oppressive humidity. The paint is blistered on the weathered door to the dormitory. It is open slightly and it's dark inside. There are a few monks walking calmly through the darkness pulling at the golden cloth of their robes. Y whispers in labored English that he is 37 years old, giggling nervously as he pauses self-consciously at trouble spots between some words. His left arm is tattooed with a large, bold dragon and a flaming spiral. He glides his right hand over the images, gently wiping away a settling fly. "One of the monks who lives inside has done the tattoos," he volunteers. "He has tattooed a few of the monks who live here. They are all Buddhist tattoos. He is old now and tattooed soldiers for protection during the war."

Monk Y.

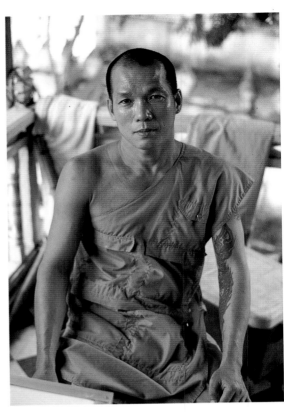

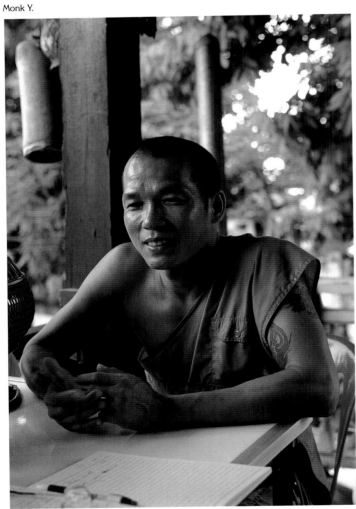

Monk Y.

"One of the monks who lives inside has done the tattoos. He has tattooed a few of the monks who live here. They are all Buddhist tattoos. He is old now and tattooed soldiers for protection during the war."

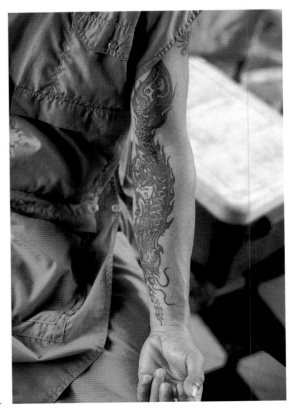

Dragon tattoo descending monk Y's left arm.

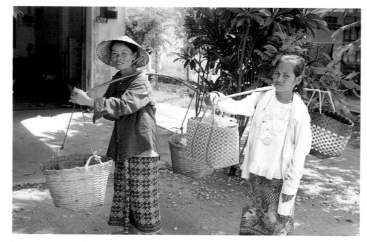

Young Lao family riding on their motorbike.

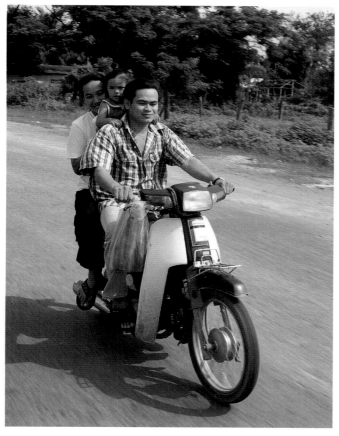

Lao women at work.

Rice cultivation.

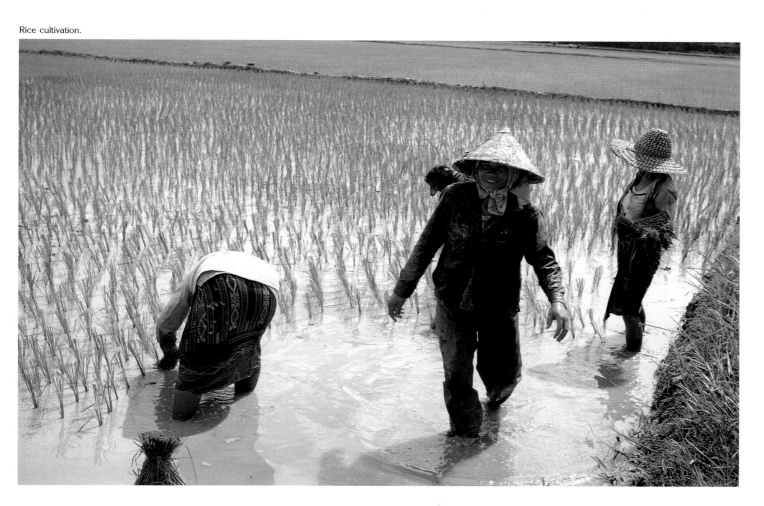

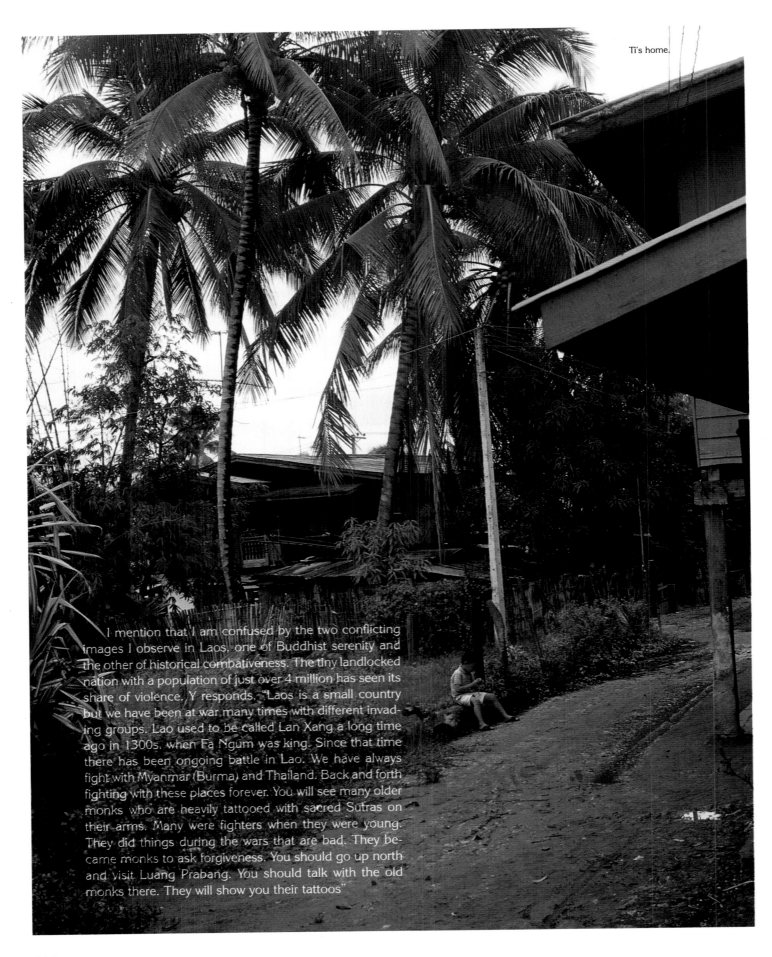

Ti's home.

I mention that I am confused by the two conflicting images I observe in Laos, one of Buddhist serenity and the other of historical combativeness. The tiny landlocked nation with a population of just over 4 million has seen its share of violence. Y responds, "Laos is a small country but we have been at war many times with different invading groups. Lao used to be called Lan Xang a long time ago in 1300s. when Fa Ngum was king. Since that time there has been ongoing battle in Lao. We have always fight with Myanmar (Burma) and Thailand. Back and forth fighting with these places forever. You will see many older monks who are heavily tattooed with sacred Sutras on their arms. Many were fighters when they were young. They did things during the wars that are bad. They became monks to ask forgiveness. You should go up north and visit Luang Prabang. You should talk with the old monks there. They will show you their tattoos"

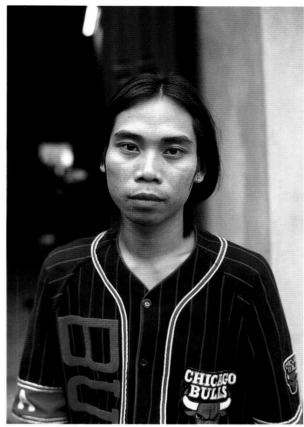

Young tattooer, Ti.

Nith brings me to visit with a young man named Ti who tattoos out of his house. We bounce along Vientiane streets past motorbike repair shops and other small businesses. There are cinder block houses surrounded with trees and bushes sprouting from red clay soil at the edge of the road. Curious dogs scramble out of their yards looking at us as we pass.

Ti is wearing an American, National Basketball Association Chicago Bulls jersey. He slips into his sandals, walks out of his small home and greets us skeptically. He has been tattooing for ten years by hand, works out of his house, but also travels to make tattoos. Nith translates as Ti describes the cultural middle ground he lives in. "I first started tattooing because I liked it and saw pictures in my head," Ti recalls. "I saw magazines with my favorite rock bands like Metallica. They were tattooed so I wanted tattoos like them."

Ti displaying his western style tattoo.

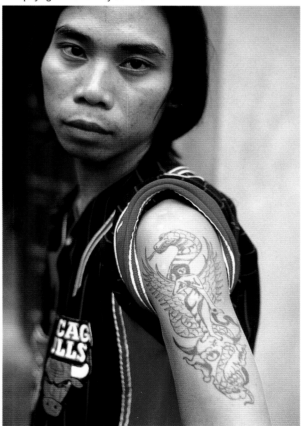

Ti obviously represents a bridge between the old culture of Laos and the steady encroachment of the West. He has a few traditional, protective symbols tattooed on his arm, but they contrast sharply with commercial, American music industry images. Because of the nature of Laotian culture today, he does not feel comfortable showing his tattoos in public. "Older people in Laos and the government do not like tattooing and these new pictures," he explains. "They feel that people with tattoos are gangsters and they do not like this. Young women in Laos do not get tattooed. If a woman has a tattoo she is either a gangster or people think she is."

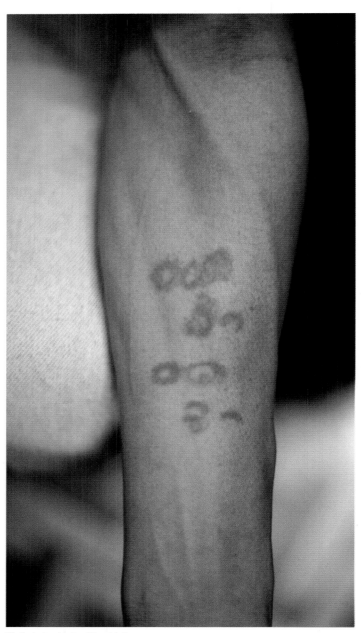

Ti displaying his traditional tattoo.

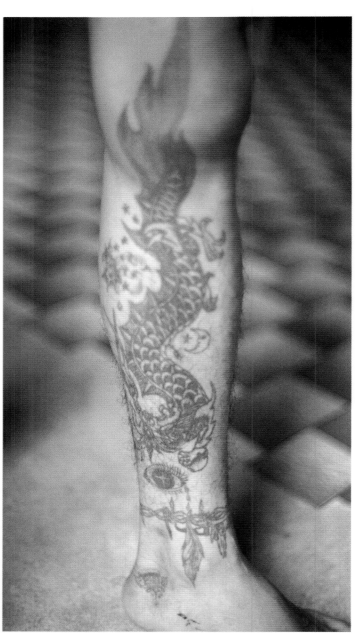

Dragon tattoo by Ti.

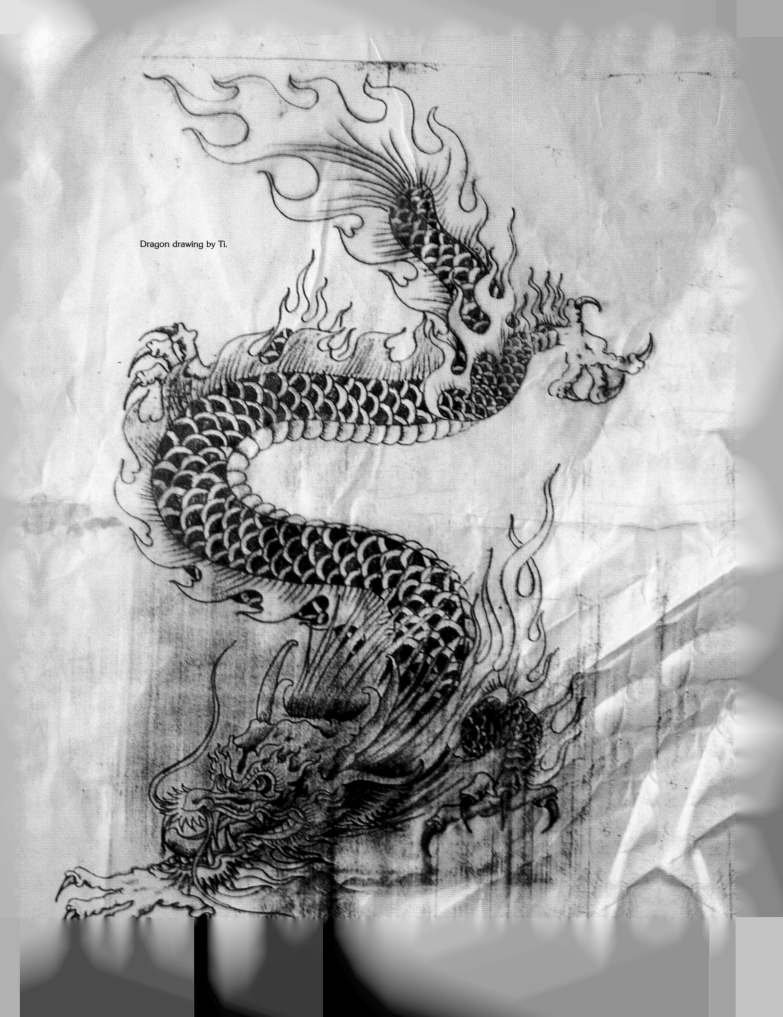

Dragon drawing by Ti.

Ti learned how to tattoo from watching the monks at Wat Vatatnoy work by hand. He studied art in school and decided to try after he saw his favorite rock stars had tattoos. "I have tattooed a lot of my male friends, but they are all hidden," he explains. "They all hide their tattoos so the government will not see them. There would be trouble if the government saw the tattoos. There are still monks up north that have old tattoos. You have to go to Luang Prabang to see them."

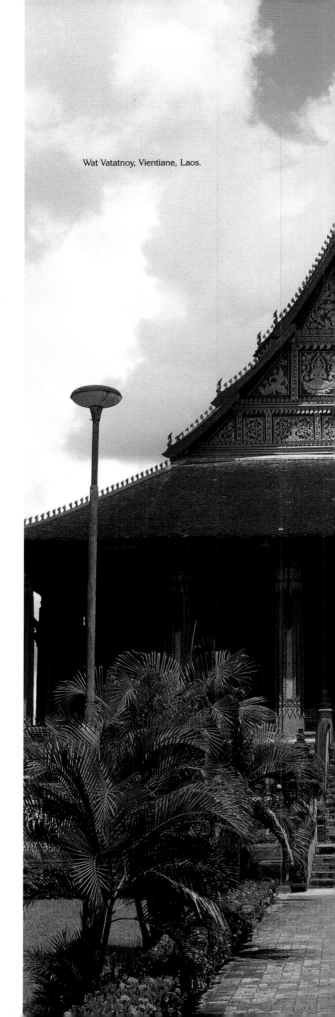

Wat Vatatnoy, Vientiane, Laos.

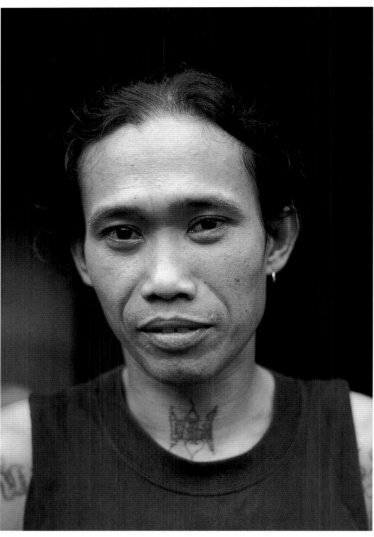

Ti's friend with traditional Lao Buddhist magical tattoo on his throat.

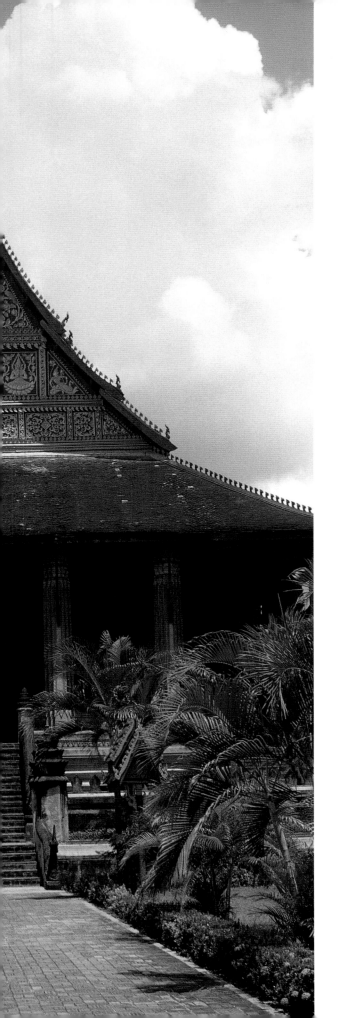

Ti's tattoo work.

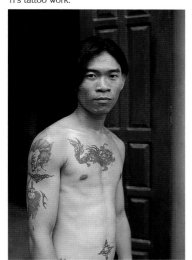

Ti's friend with Lao Buddhist magical tattoos.

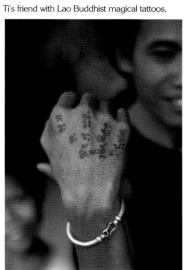

Ti's tattoo work.

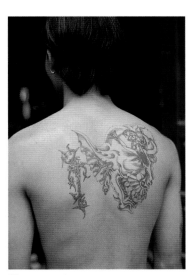

Ti's friend with Buddhist magical tattoos.

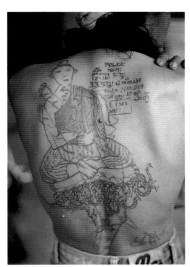

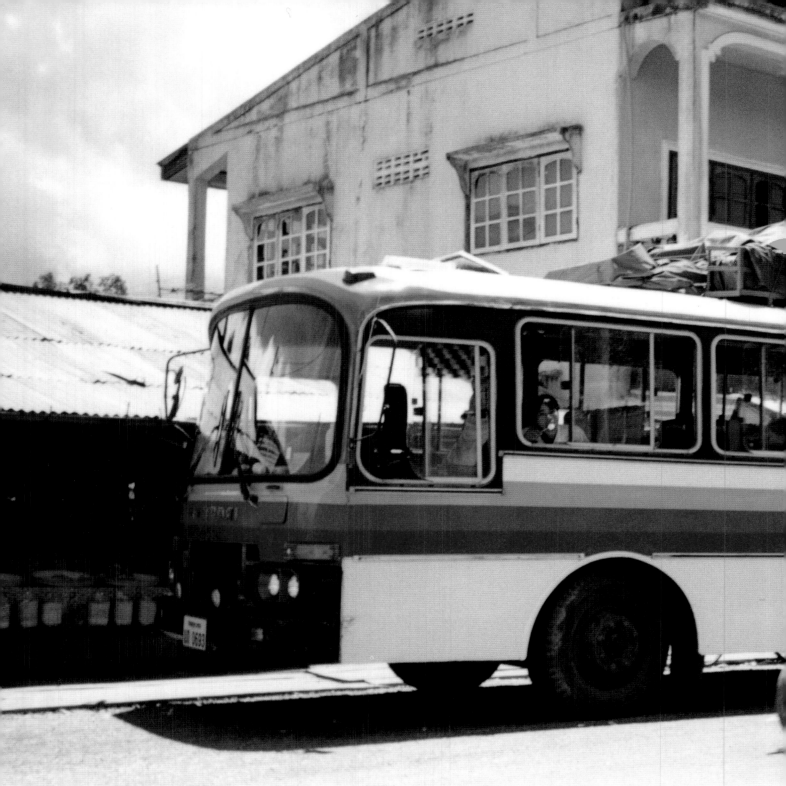

The bus to Luang Prabang sits in front of the ticket booth at the hot and dusty Vientiane bus depot. Lao families mill around in the chaos, passing huge burlap wrapped boxes and objects up to the driver who is lashing it all onto the roof. The bus rocks from side to side as the driver shifts the heap around. Passengers prepare for the 17-hour journey, purchasing an assortment of hand cooked food from young women carrying sacks around their shoulders. All loaded, the interior of the bus smells like an exotic restaurant as it pulls out, headed towards the distant, 9000-foot mountains. As we climb into the green foothills, the road switchbacks through dangerous narrow passes with panoramic views of huge, ancient mountains covered with lush stands of old teak. Hungry passengers stare out the window eating lychee nuts and wild cucumber; the driver blasts his air horn to warn oncoming vehicles of our approach. Women walking along the road carry heavy bundles on their back and step aside as we pass. They are dressed traditionally in ankle-length sarongs with stripes of black, blue, gold and maroon.

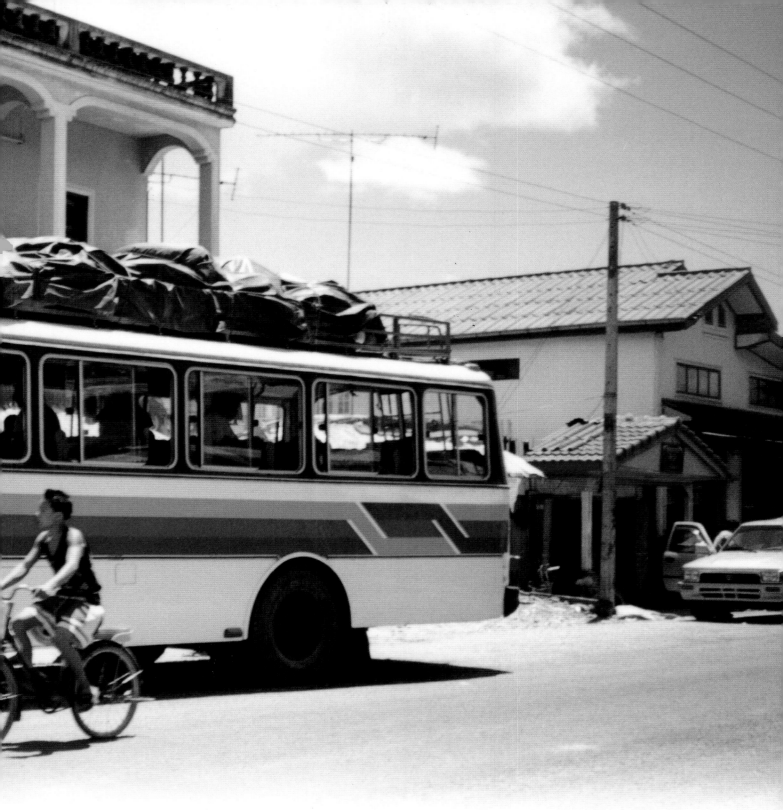

Bus to Luang Prabang, Laos.

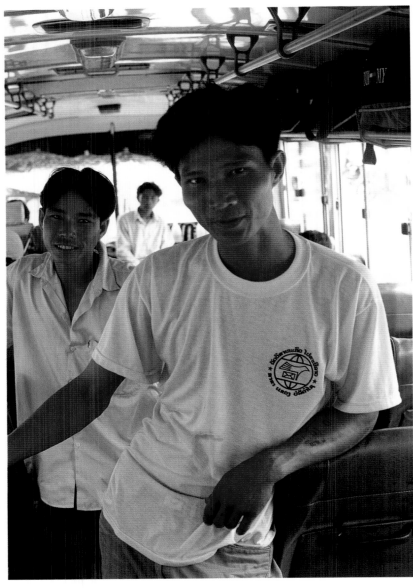

Passenger on Luang Prabang bus with tattoo received in Lao prison.

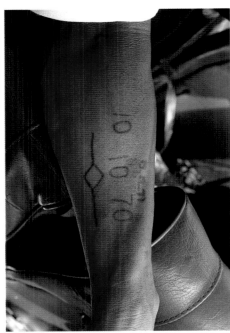

Lao prison tattoo.

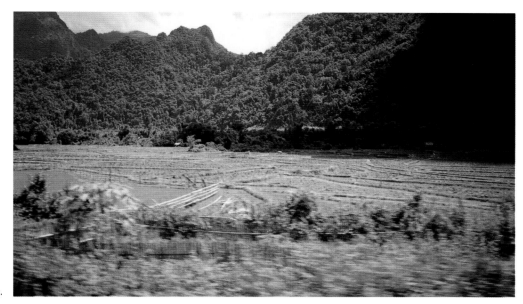

Lao countryside on trip to Luang Prabang.

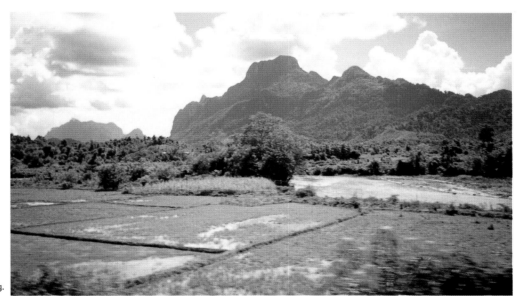

Lao countryside on trip to Luang Prabang.

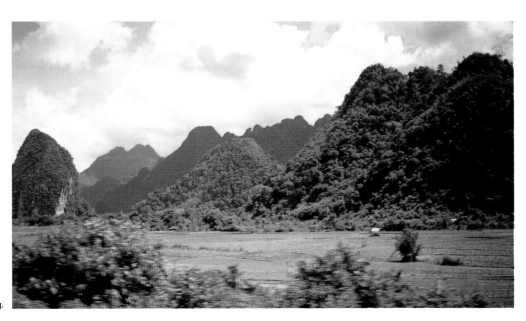

Lao mountains on trip to Luang Prabang.

The ancient Lao capital Luang Prabang is situated high on a peninsula where the Man Khan and Mekong rivers meet. There are over 30 ancient temples that have survived the trial of time since the fourteenth century. Hundreds of saffron robed Buddhist monks shuffle around the quiet streets under sunshade umbrellas.

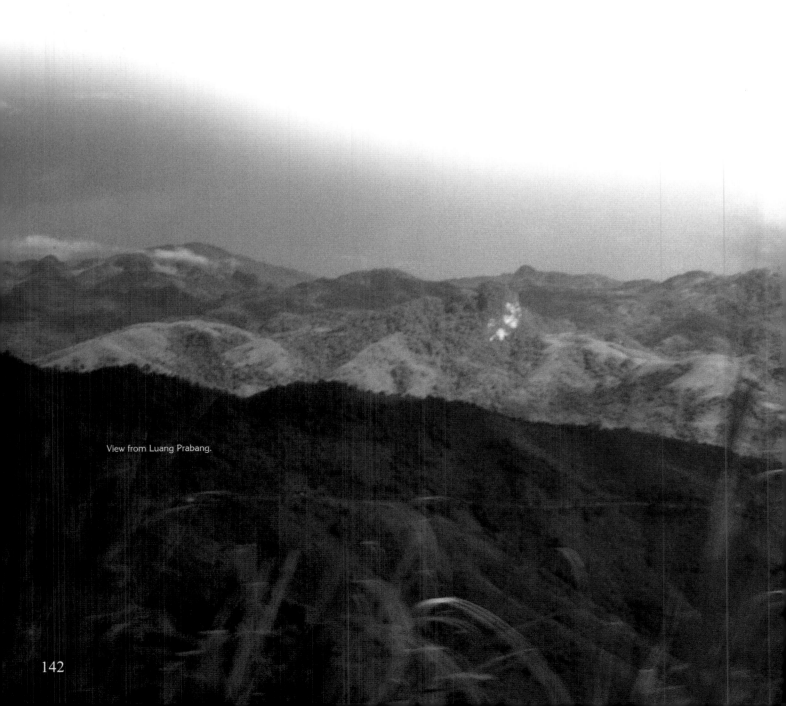

View from Luang Prabang.

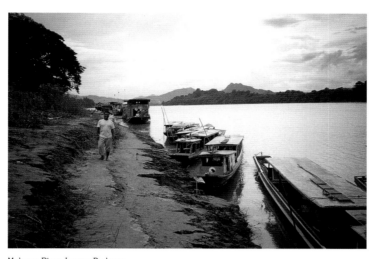
Mekong River, Luang Prabang.

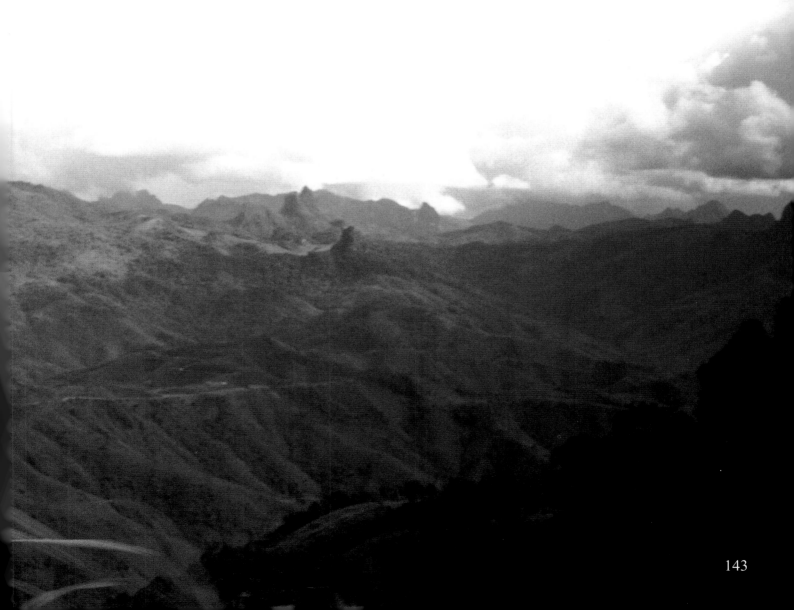

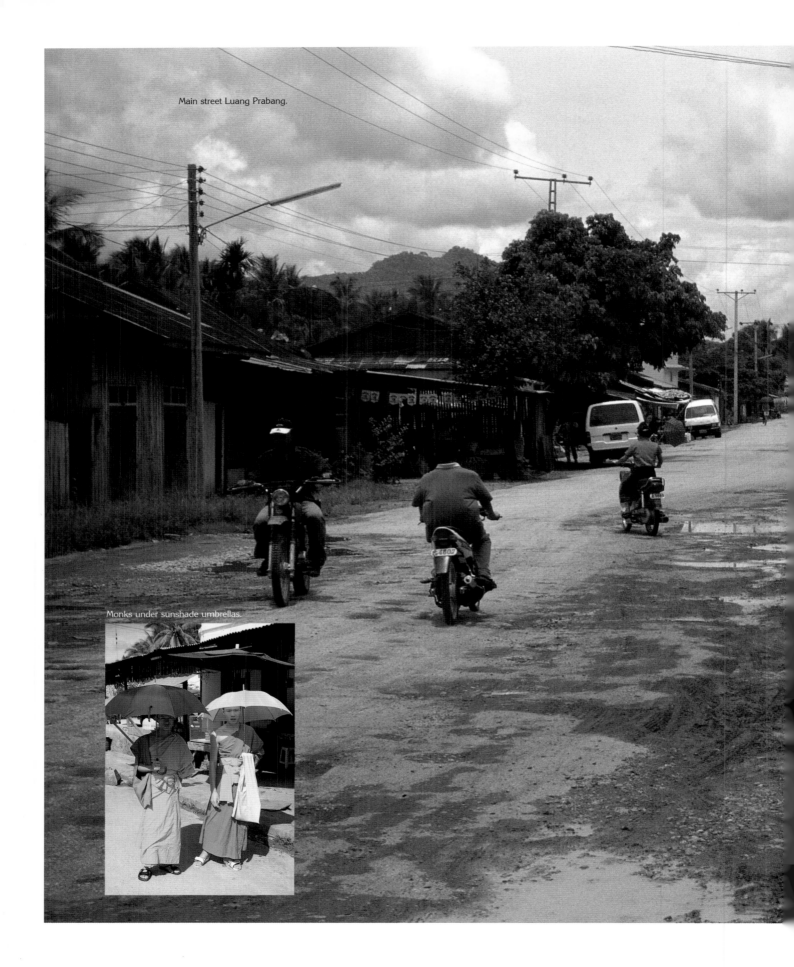

Main street Luang Prabang.

Monks under sunshade umbrellas.

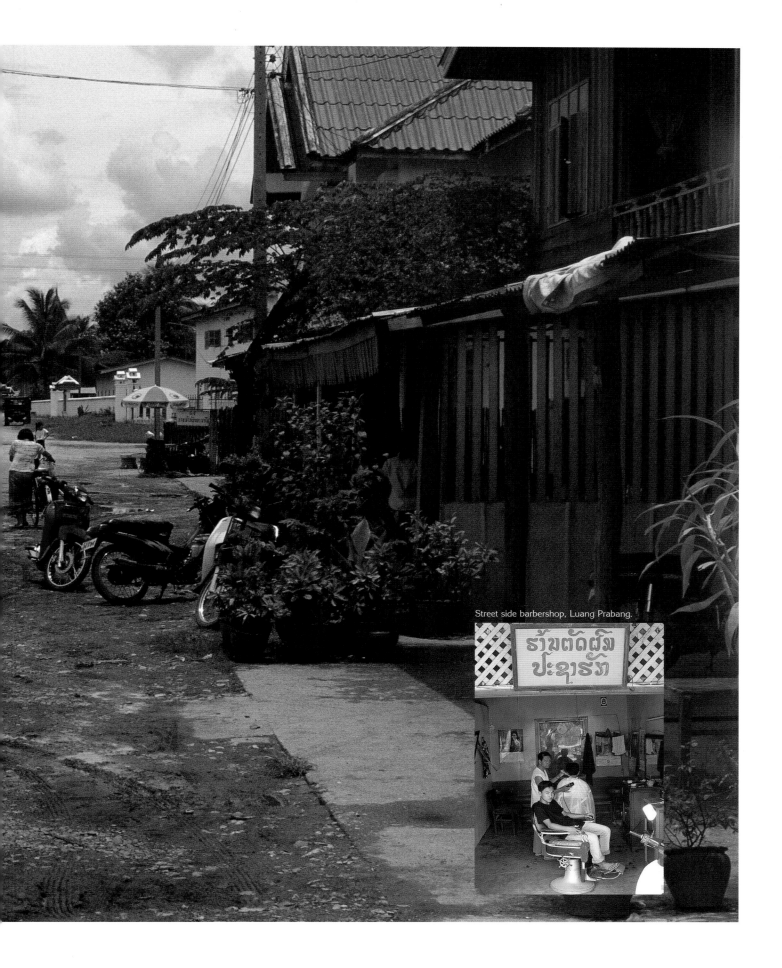

Street side barbershop, Luang Prabang.

At a street-side shop a young man named Seangphone shows me a magical symbol his grandmother encouraged him to have tattooed on his shoulder. He chuckles when he tells me it is meant to protect him from bullets, telling me he got it partly to appease his traditionally minded grandmother and partly because he believes in its power. He tells me that as a boy he became a novice monk in an effort to receive an education and learn English. He knows many of the senior monks in Luang Prabang who are tattooed and graciously volunteers to introduce me to them.

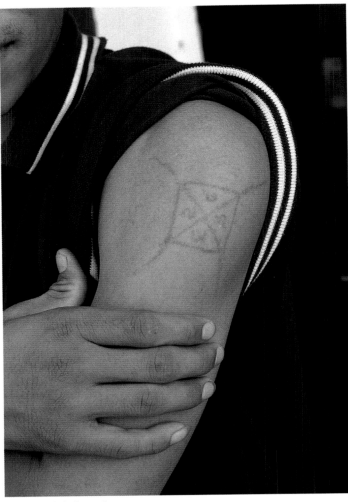

Seangphone's bulletproof tattoo.

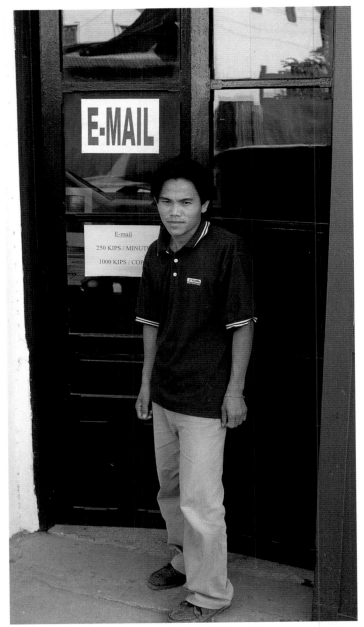

Seangphone.

146

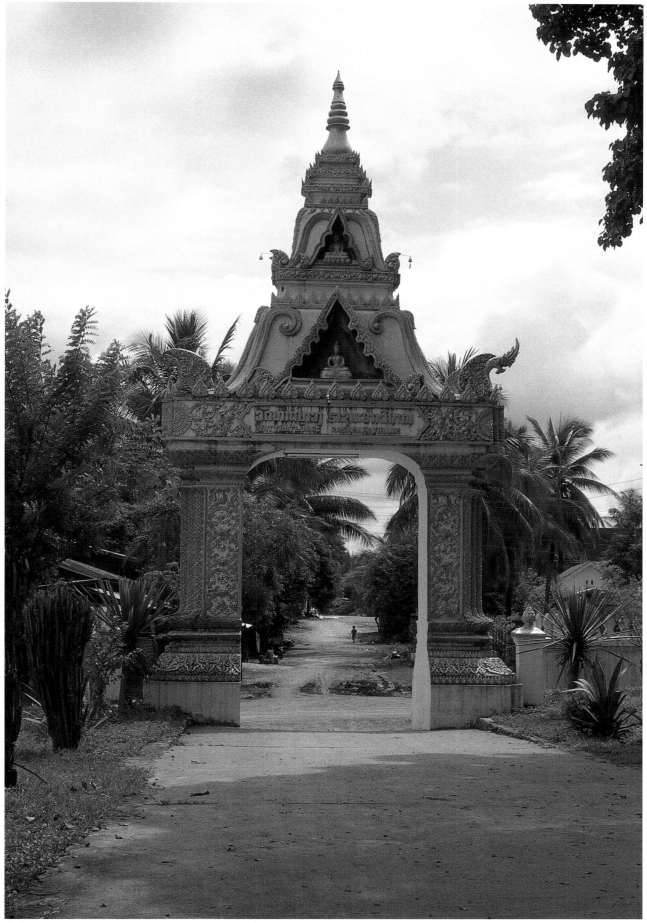

Vat Manorom.

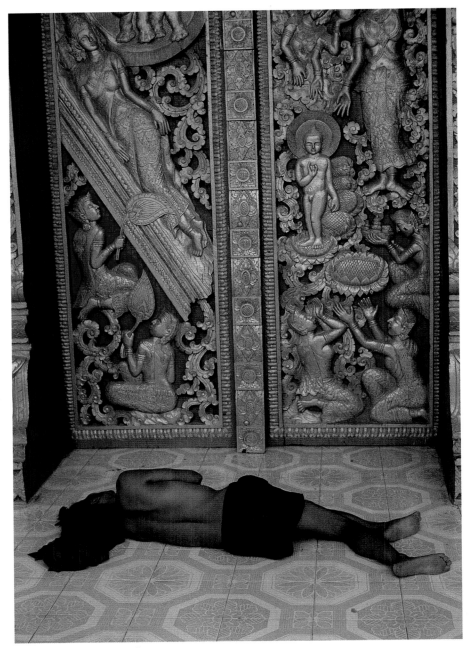

Young boy sleeping at temple door.

We enter Vat Manorom and Seang introduces me to a young novice monk named Bounkhain who will help to introduce me to the older monks. He will also explain the fundamentals of Theravada Buddhism in Indochina, which in my mind is crucial to understanding why people here get tattooed. We talk with Bounk at the feet of a huge Buddha erected in 1371 in the main altar room that was built in 1363. The air is thick with incense smoke coming from smaller secondary altars stepped off below the great Buddha. Several curious, young novice monks gather near. The young boys are very shy and withdrawn. They sit cross-legged a safe distance away, avoiding eye contact.

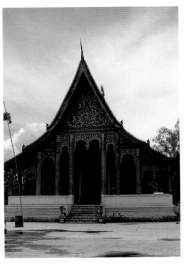

Vat Manorom.

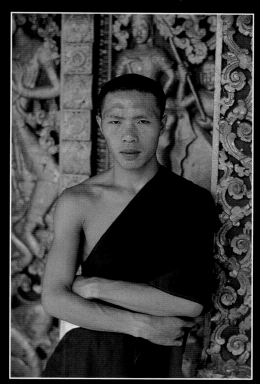

Novice monk Bounkhain.

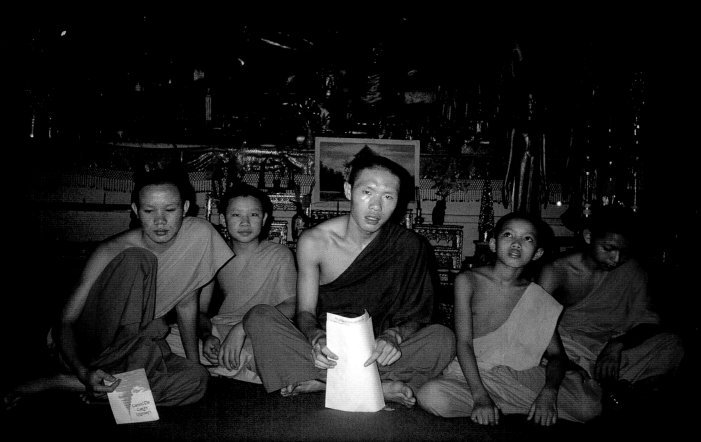

Monk Bounk with students.

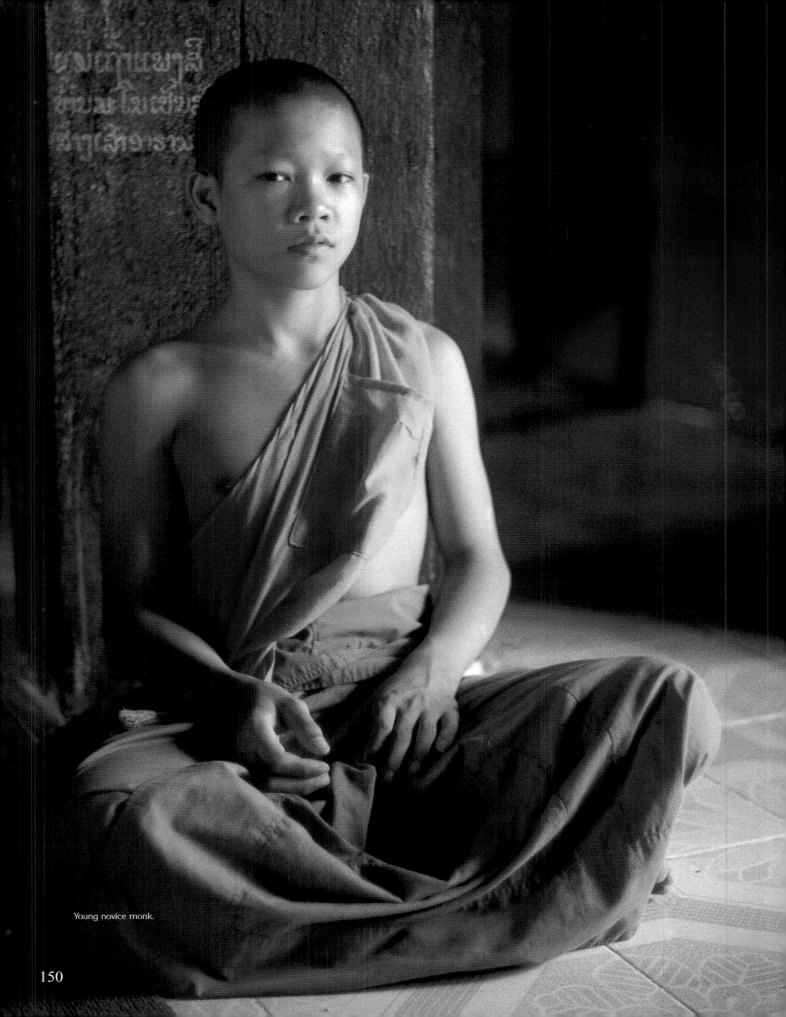

Young novice monk.

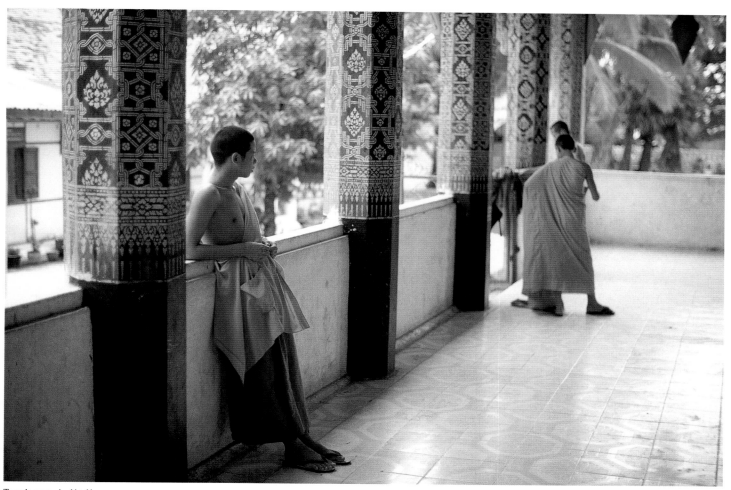

Temple veranda, Vat Manorom.

Bounk begins saying, "I came from a small village 350 km from here in northern Lao that had no schools." He speaks deliberately, working at the correct pronunciation of each word. "There are very few schools in northern villages. Young boys become novices at 12 to 19 years old. When they are 20 they become a monk. They grow rice in my village. My family works on a farm. I am from the Chat tribal group. In the northern villages, people respect the spirits of nature, tree spirits, spirits of the rocks."

"I became a novice monk to learn. I study Buddhism, the mathematics, English for composition to teach visitors about history of this Wat. The Sak (tattoos) you will see on the older monks here and at other Wats have to do with the fighting. Many people in Lao have Sak for fighting and war. Old people and traditional hill tribe people have Sak for fighting. Now tattoos are not common. People find it too painful today."

Bounk continues, talking about the different schools of Buddhism found in Indochina and their influence on tattoo practices in the region. "Buddhism first entered Indochina in two parts," Bounk explains. "During the early millennia of our time scholars from India taught the Mahayana form of Buddhism and it reached the height of devotion in the twelfth and thirteenth centuries. Then in the fourteenth century a second wave of Buddhism, Theravada thought, entered from China. Today, the people of Indochina are Theravada Buddhists.

"The old Mahayana school teaches group salvation. It is possible for all people to reach enlightenment. Theravada Buddhism teaches enlightenment is reserved solely for a select few scholars and monks. It is called the teaching of elders. Mahayana teaches the Bodhisattva or teacher is an important figure. The Bodhisattva is unique to Mahayana. The Bodhisattva is a soul who has already reach the enlightenment, but through compassion stays and helps all people on earth to reach enlightenment."

I ask Bounk if he feels that tattooing has a purpose in Indochina because of the limitation of the Theravada form. If only a few elder, scholarly monks are chosen for enlightenment, what about everybody else? What can they do? Is this tattoo tradition a way to insure protection and salvation even if they are not a chosen person? Bounk thinks for a minute and says, "There are old religions of superstition and animism in Indochina. They are older than the Buddhism but they are still here underneath everything for people. The tattoos are a combination of everything. People try to make everything work good."

Bounk leads us out of the altar building towards a building where the monks live. We enter a very humble series of rooms where senior monks are sleeping in the incredible mid-morning heat and humidity. The tables and chairs look rough and hand-hewn. There are fabric tapestries hanging loosely on the walls that have images of the Buddha sitting and meditating. Bounk asks me

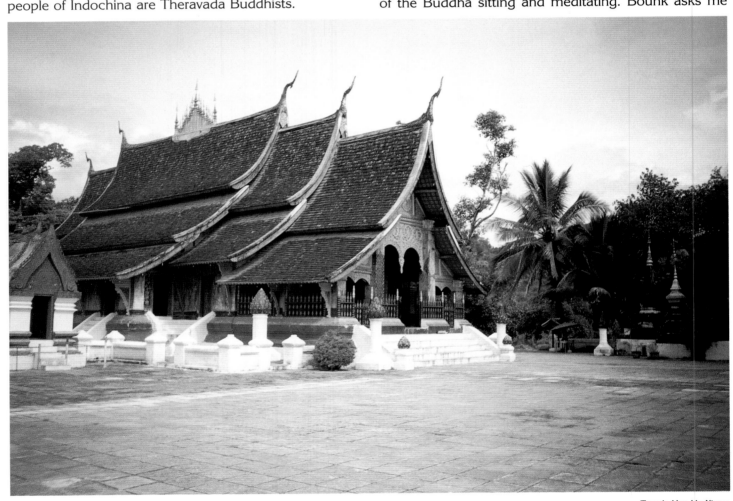

Temple Hoc Ho Xieng.

152

not to photograph the tapestries. One by one Bounk gently shakes each monk's shoulders and awakens them. They rise gently, rub their eyes and look perplexed to see me. Khampeo, the senior monk of the temple is 65 years old. He was tattooed at 18 with Buddhist sutras down his arms that were meant to protect him. Bounk awakens a monk named Vanh, which means One. He is 68 years old and was tattooed when he was 7 years old. Both men were soldiers fighting for Lao independence in the 1950s. "These are the last examples of this type of magic tattooing," Bounk says as the monks search the shelves near their beds for a pack of cigarettes. "The monks are tattooed with the Thom Buddhist language. It was used in former times before the standardization of Lao 800 years ago. When you see the text it is always justified evenly on both the right and left margins. Thom was used by monks to communicate amongst themselves. It is thought to be an offshoot of Sanskrit. Both monks believe their tattoos saved them during the fight for independence. The sutras are a Buddhist blessing with a strong meaning."

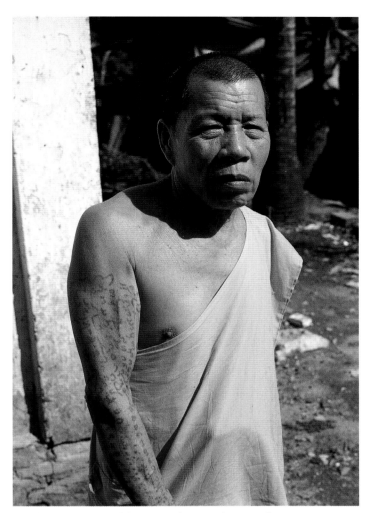

Monk Khampeo with sacred Sutra tattoos he received to protect him.

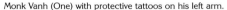

Monk Vanh (One) with protective tattoos on his left arm.

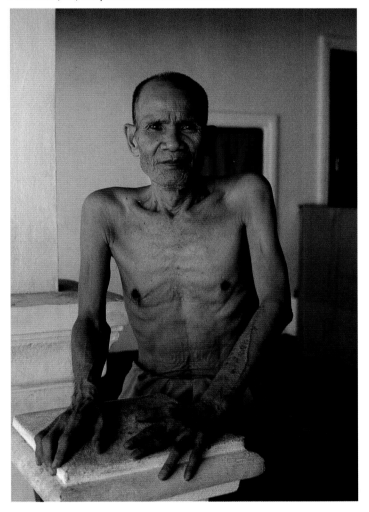

"There are old religions of superstition and animism in Indochina. They are older than the Buddhism but they are still here underneath everything for people. The tattoos are a combination of everything. People try to make everything work good."

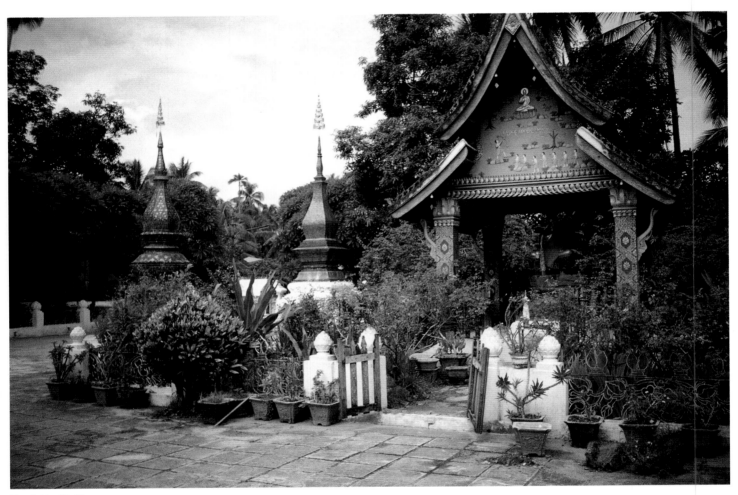

Temple Hoc Ho Xieng.

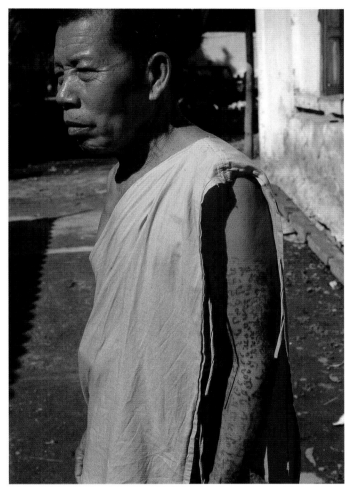

Monk Khampeo with sacred Sutra tattoos.

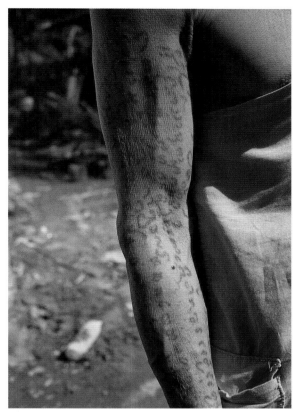

Close-up of monk Khampeo's tattoos.

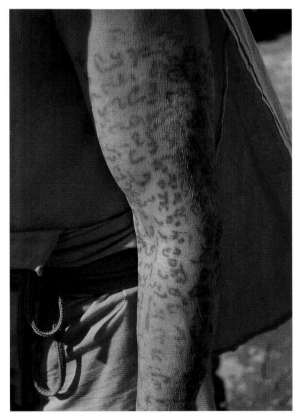

Close-up of monk Khampeo's tattoos.

Seang wants me to meet a monk named Souk and drives me to a nearby temple called Hoc Ho Xieng where he lived as a novice for several years. We take off our shoes and walk into a dark altar chapel where there are several monks sleeping on the red carpeted floor in their saffron robes. The tall walls have very old peeling frescos painted on them and there are dozens of 6-inch square, rectangular insets that have miniature Buddha figurines in them. Monk Souk is curled up on the floor at the foot of a large Buddha that is 600 years old. As Seang shakes the monk into consciousness, I am told he is 105 years old and I cringe as he pops up looking at me. There is both a resiliency and fragility to Monk Souk. He sits and stares at me, blinking his deep-set heavy-lidded eyes, and asks Seang who I am and where I came from. Seang laughs and explains why I am here and Souk suggests that we go out front where the light is better. Souk explains that he has been a monk for 80 or more years and asks if I have any cigarettes. As a young man he left the monkhood for 3 or 4 years and fought for Lao independence. He then reentered the monkhood to atone for his actions when he was a soldier. The magical phrases which run down his arm, were tattooed by monks to protect him from guns and bullets. The phrases were taken from ancient Buddhist texts.

Magical cloth from temple with tattoo designs.

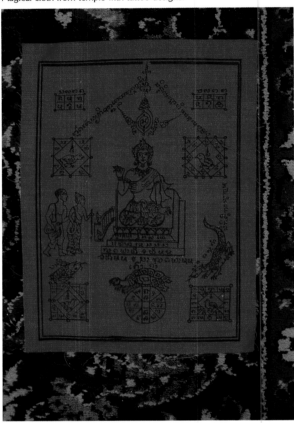

Monk Souk.

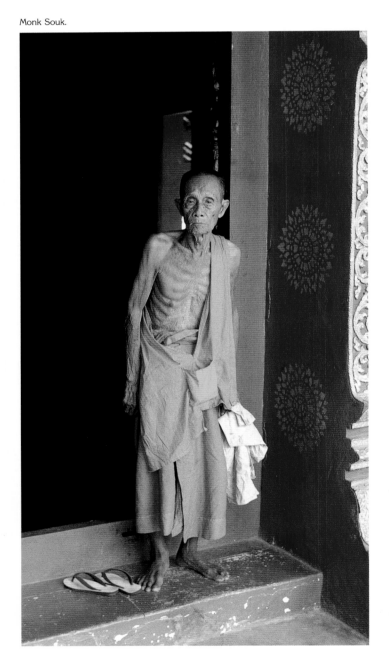

Monk Souk's protective tattoos.

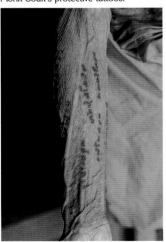

Monk Souk's protective tattoos.

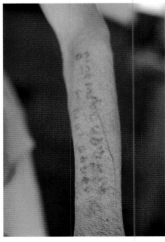

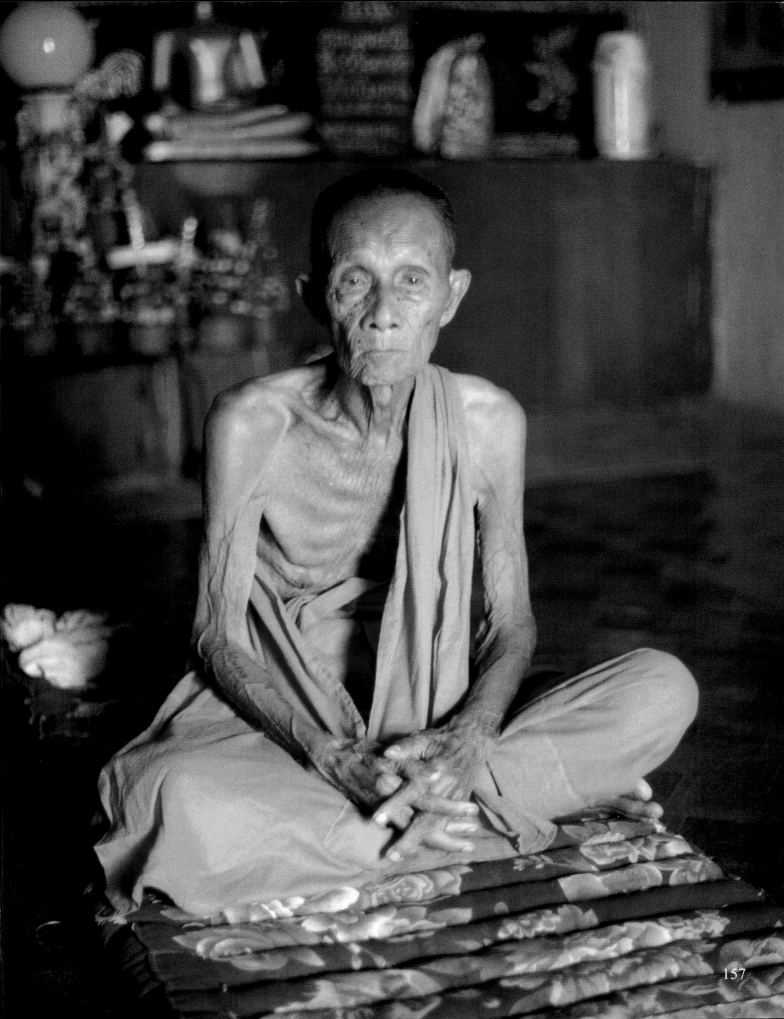

There is a 98-year-old man from the Leu hill tribe who Seang feels is important for me to meet. He lives in the Panom village, which is 3 miles outside Luang Prabang. We drive towards the surrounding hills in a Tuk-Tuk, bouncing down red dirt roads that cut through heavy tropical forest. The old man is sitting in front of his modest home watching his granddaughter working at her large handloom. Lao women are known for their exact and meticulous loom work.

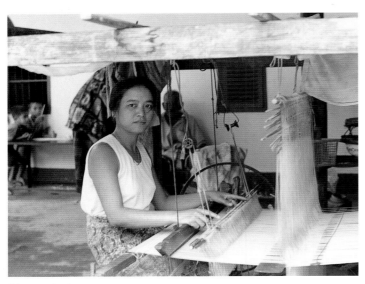

Woman at her loom.

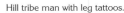

Hill tribe man with leg tattoos.

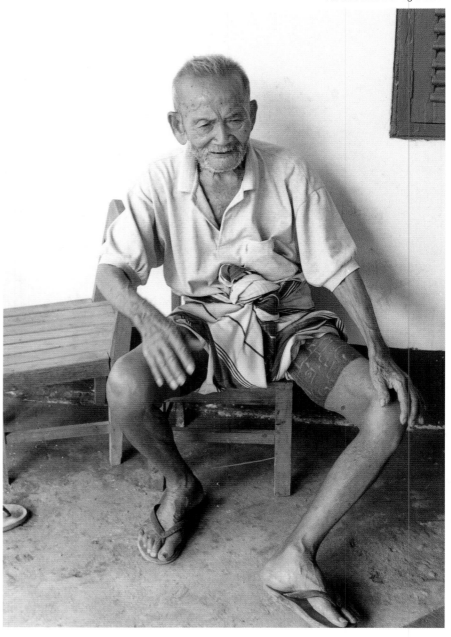

As the young woman pulls at her loom, the old man shows me his impressive tribal leg tattoos. He motions at his large, black spiral designs chopping at them with his palm and then waves off his chopping to say that he can not be cut there. He tells me through Seang that old men tattooed him in his village before he went off to fight. The tattooing was done by hand with crude metal needles and it was very painful. It was like a test, to see if the young men getting tattooed could withstand the pain. Fighting was very challenging and the pain of the tattoo prepared them for fighting in the jungle, which is very dangerous. He roamed the jungle for months with his comrades, there was little food and they had to watch out for wild animals that would try to attack them. They had few guns and little ammunition. When they found the enemy they would wait and follow them the way a tiger would hunt. They would wait for the right time and then attack at night and cut everybody's throat in their sleep. They knew the jungle better than the enemy and it helped them to find them and kill them. They would prop the bodies up against trees so they would be devoured by animals. When the enemy found the torn-apart bodies of their comrades it destroyed their spirit.

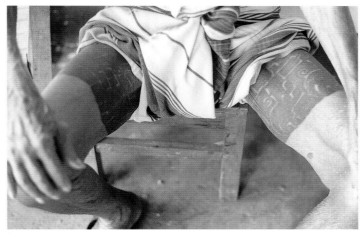

Leg tattoos.

The spiral designs are old and powerful. The design is magical and works against evil; it has been a part of the art for a long time. Seang tells me that the hill tribe man fought in the war against the French and Japanese. Like the monks, his tattoos are protective. He is one of the few remaining men who have these types of tattoos. There was a time when the surrounding hills had many tattooed men but they are all gone now.

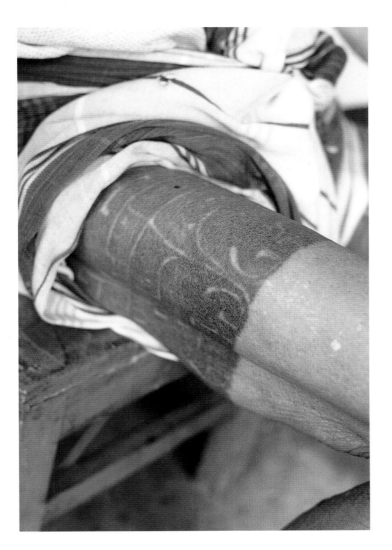

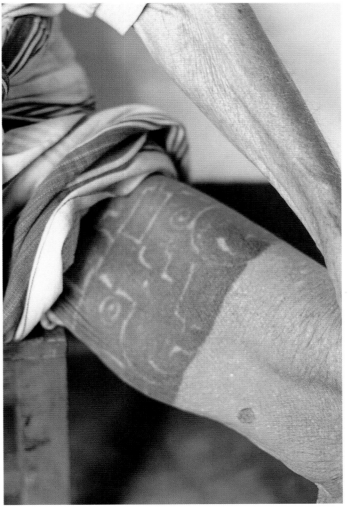

POSTSCRIPT

Today in the West, particularly among young adults, interest about the art form of tattooing has exploded. Young women and men who want to be in touch with the trends of their time, feel compelled to wear some kind of tattooed mark. The permanent ink in their skin feels culturally relevant and there is a momentary thrill as tenets are challenged. For a percentage of hard-core enthusiasts an industry and lifestyle has taken shape in recent years. It has formalized around a post-modern body aesthetic that exists in a secular, sub-cultural vacuum for the most part. People in this western tattoo community read their own magazines, attend an assortment of their own conventions and communicate about their art using a specialized, nuanced vocabulary. Beyond this, for the majority of people who get tattooed very human questions are posed and possibly answered.

Throughout my stay in Indochina, as I learned about the tattooing there, I was struck by similarities and differences between what I was observing and what exists in the West. Unlike the West, tattoos in Indochina do not exist in a secular subcultural vacuum. The tattoos and designs of Indochina are a part of a complete, mainstream historical package. They exist within the overall context of people's lives. This is why I have included so many supporting images in this book. In Indochina, tattoos are a part of what goes on there. As the values of modernization have gained precedence, enforced by strict political ideology or inspired by blatant western influence, the sense of resolve about tattoo traditions may be changing but it remains.

The older men I talked with displayed their tattoos with pride and seriousness. It described their obvious connection to a historical process and a powerful belief system that are thousands of years old. The young people I talked with throughout the region proudly displayed their new Western style tattoos as examples of global sophistication but also showed me their traditional tattoos with self-respect. During the planning stage of this project the cultural institutions I contacted wondered suspiciously why I was bothering. There was an obvious sensitivity to the issue of an outsider from the West snooping into private information, possibly mischaracterizing it and imposing significance onto people. A natural reaction in the post-colonial world. There are serious issues of globalization, development and self-preservation in the region that take precedence.

Wherever I went I always connected with people with tattoos. They saw mine and immediately showed me theirs. There was a genuine sense of curiosity, camaraderie and pride that opened doors for me. Whether it was Tuk-tuk men in Bangkok, ex-Khmer Rouge soldiers in Cambodia, or Buddhist priests in Laos, the common denominator of being tattooed broke the ice and transcended class, race, and political ideology. There is something about people putting marks onto themselves that dives to the core of the frail human condition. The impulse reveals basic unknowns about our lives that nag at us and refuse to leave us alone. As I talked with people, photographed and took notes I was inspired by the conversations and realized that even in our rapidly changing world, our differences are dwarfed by what we all have in common.